D1086232

Leaders and Followers: A Psychiatric Perspective on Religious Cults

Middlesex County College
Library, Edison, NJ 08818

Committee on Psychiatry and Religion
Group for the Advancement of Psychiatry

Richard C. Lewis, New Haven, CT, *Chairperson*
Naleen N. Andrade, Honolulu, HI
Keith G. Meador, Nashville, TN
Abigail R. Ostow, Belmont, MA
Sally K. Severino, White Plains, NY
Clyde R. Snyder, Fayetteville, NC
Edwin R. Wallace IV, Augusta, GA

Albert J. Lubin, Woodside, CA, *Former Chairperson*
Sidney Furst, Bronx, NY, *Former Member*
Mortimer Ostow, Bronx, NY, *Former Member*

Leaders and Followers: A Psychiatric Perspective on Religious Cults

Formulated by the Committee on
Psychiatry and Religion

Group for the Advancement of Psychiatry

Report No. 132

Published by

Washington, DC
London, England

Copyright © 1992 Group for the Advancement of Psychiatry.
ALL RIGHTS RESERVED
Manufactured in the United States of America on acid-free paper.
94 93 92 91 4 3 2 1
Published by American Psychiatric Press, Inc., 1400 K Street, N.W.,
Washington, DC 20005.

Library of Congress Cataloging-in-Publication Data

Leaders and followers : a psychiatric perspective on religious cults /
formulated by the Committee on Psychiatry and Religion, Group
for the Advancement of Psychiatry
    p. cm. -- (Report ; no. 132)
    Includes bibliographical references
    ISBN 0-87318-200-6 (alk. paper)
    1. Cults--United States--Psychology. 2. Cults--Dead Sea Region (Is-
rael and Jordan)--Psychology--History. 3. Psychiatry and religion. I.
Group for the Advancement of Psychiatry. Committee on Psychiatry
and Religion. II. Series: Report (Group for the Advancement of Psychiatry : 1984) ; no. 132.
RC321.G7 no. 132
[BP603]
616.89s--dc20
[291'.0973]   91-20979
                                                                        CIP

British Cataloguing in Publication Data

A CIP record is available from the British Library.

Contents

Preface

You have noticed that the human being is a curiosity. In times past he has had (and worn out and flung away) hundreds and hundreds of religions, and launches not fewer than three new ones every year. I could enlarge that number and still be within the facts.

Mark Twain, *Letters From the Earth*

Numerous disturbing reports by parents, psychotherapists and clergy, as well as newspaper and magazine articles declaiming the evils of religious cults motivated the Committee on Psychiatry and Religion to undertake this study. For the most part, these were stories about heinous activities and harmful effects on cult followers. The possibility of some beneficial effect was rarely considered. At the outset we expected to find rampant psychopathology in the cult leaders and in those who followed them. In due course, we learned that cults vary greatly in composition, structure, and practices. Some pose a serious threat to their followers; others may serve a more benign, if usually transient, purpose for youths with certain psychological needs. Though cult membership is generally a maladaptive response to these needs, most cults were neither all good nor all bad. In deciding on an appropriate response to the phenomenon of the cults, one must carefully consider the conflict between the rights of individuals to freely exercise their religious beliefs, and the need of society to protect its members against the serious dangers that some cults can pose. Thus, we felt we could not develop a position on the cults that was appropriate to all situations.

Any analysis of the cults is hampered by a lack of information. Secretiveness, inaccessibility to dialogue, and disaffiliation from mainline denominations no doubt contribute to public suspicion of the cults and to the tendency to interpret their deviance as deviousness. Such judgments may be based on emotional response rather than reasoned evaluation.

Information about the beliefs, rites, and organization of the "new religions" is difficult to obtain. These groups are isolated from the surrounding community. They may avoid contact with theological seminaries or be refused membership in ministerial associations. Their recent origin prohibits accumulation of reliable history or knowledge about their aims and ways. Sometimes members are sworn to secrecy, and some seem to be deliberately inarticulate about their tenets. Authoritarian leadership tends to resist public accountability. Some leaders have been clearly fraudulent. Some have made a litigious response to attempts to hold them accountable to the public. Some groups are torn by inner strife that hampers reporting. Some groups are neither shy nor secretive about their recruitment efforts; they issue magazines and run membership training programs. However, there may be a significant discrepancy between the group's image as held out to the prospective recruit, and the realities of day to day life within the cult.

The Committee on Psychiatry and Religion of the American Psychiatric Association has also recently studied cults and new religious movements and has published a report on the subject. This group concluded that there were legitimate differences of opinion among those who study the cults, and that no clear recommendations could be made about how to deal with the cults and their members. The report presented several different papers representing a variety of viewpoints and invited the reader to draw his own conclusions.

We feel that any sort of a preconceived judgment or stance could seriously impair meaningful communication between cult members and those family and friends "outside" who would reach them. While we do not attempt to justify or defend cults, neither do we mean to add to the wealth of literature that decries them. Instead, we have tried to generate a perspective from which an individual and the cult he or she follows can be more rationally evaluated; with the understanding so gained, more informed recommendations can be made. We hope that this sort of study will be useful to parents, teachers, therapists, and any others dealing with prospective, current, and former cult members. Enhanced understanding of the psychological needs of the cults' "victims" might also inform the efforts of mainstream organizations to constructively assist our youth in the developmental tasks facing them.

We include in our report a description of some American cults and a more detailed look at an ancient sect. There has been an apparent increase in cults and cult membership during the past 20 years, and because of this, some assume that cults are a new phenomenon. In fact, cults have been with us as long as there has been organized religion. Their popularity seems to increase with certain kinds of social stress, when fears and uncertainties are not adequately answered by more mainstream social organizations.

References

Galanter M (ed): Cults and New Religious Movements. Washington, DC, American Psychiatric Association, 1989

Bordewich FM: Colorado's Thriving Cults. New York Times Magazine, May 1, 1988, pp 39–44

Corporate Mind Control. Newsweek, May 4, 1987, pp 38–39

Chapter 1

Definitions

The term "cult" is frequently applied to a wide range of groups—political, therapeutic, magical, even scientific. Those who use the term generally imply that the group is irrational in its beliefs and dogmatically led by a charismatic, possibly unscrupulous leader. In this sense, the name cult can be applied to holistic medicine groups, health food enthusiasts, astrologers, EST, Neo-Nazis, White Supremacists, and the Arkansas Survivalists among others. Followers of the "New Age" philosophy are increasing in number and can currently be found among the business, entertainment, political, and military communities. One critic believes them to be the most powerful social force in the country today (see, for example, Bordewich 1988).

While obviously important, these groups differ from the religious cults that we have studied in that they are largely composed of the middle-aged, rather than youth, and their members are generally more integrated into secular society, living and working outside of the cult. The psychology and motivations of these followers are somewhat different from those of youth in religious cults and will not be dealt with in our report.

Classically, the term "cult" has applied to various eccentric forms of religious worship and the groups that practice them. During the past 20 years, however, the word has taken on a pejorative meaning and generally implies that the group is suspect. Critics use the term to describe groups they regard as false, dishonorable, and predatory, and apply it to nonreligious groups that are seen as doctrinaire and extreme. It can be said that one person's religion is another person's cult. In this report, we restrict usage of the term "cult" to groups that claim a religious or spiritual foun-

1

dation, and we distinguish these cults from social groups, political groups, and other groups that claim to offer improvement of body or mind and that have similar characteristics. The latter may be called "cultlike."

"Religions" Versus "Cults"

The three major Western faiths—Judaism, Catholicism, and Protestantism—have at times resorted to banning, shunning, ostracizing, and persecuting "cult" members—that is, members of groups that deviate from the party line—presumably in order to maintain purity of belief, specificity of ritual, propriety of conduct, or the prerogatives of priestly power. The rationale for such violent opposition has often been overstated, and similarities between established denominations and some of the cults have been ignored. Many "odd" traits of cultic religion can be seen as variations on established religious practice. By the same token, members of religious organizations commonly labeled cults call their organizations religions. Clearly, the name "cult" can be used in an arbitrary and controversial manner.

In attempting to make the term more precise, a *cult* has been defined as a group that follows a dominant leader who claims to be or is regarded by followers as infallible and divine. Group membership is contingent upon acceptance of the leader's claims and loyal obedience to his commands (Jewish Community Council of Philadelphia 1978). This definition can be applied to some generally accepted religions and is not definitive. In fact, many religions were regarded as cults at their inception and only achieved status as religions after they had attracted many followers over a long period of time.

Time and acceptance, then, are necessary, for a cult to become a generally accepted religion. Melton (1984) has called cults "first generation religions." Hence, a cult may be considered a stage in the formation of a religion, albeit a religion that may not come to fruition. Sometimes cults are co-opted into existing religions.

Willa Appel (1983) lists traits that she considered common to major American cults:

- authoritarian leadership and organization
- regimentation of members
- renunciation of the world

- doctrinaire belief that the cult has superior access to ultimate truth
- attitude of moral superiority
- contempt for secular laws
- rigid thought patterns
- low regard for individuals.

As already suggested, many of these traits are not unique to cults but are conspicuous in churches that have been part of American culture since colonial times. A similar criticism may be made of the definition of Philip Cushman (1984). He defines a cult as a group that

- is controlled by a charismatic leader who is thought to be God or carries an exclusive message from God,
- fosters the idea that there is only one correct belief and one correct practice,
- demands unquestioning obedience and loyalty to its totalitarian methods,
- uses methods of mind control,
- uses deception when recruiting,
- systematically exploits members' labor and finances, and attacks or abandons members who disagree or leave the group.

"Cults" and "Sects"

So far we have not attempted to distinguish cults from sects. Current usage seems to label groups that define themselves as dissidents within particular religions as sects, and those that define themselves by creating or pursuing alien forms of worship as cults. In the discussion that follows we will distinguish between centripetal dissidents, who see themselves as restoring an actual or hypothetical original state, and centrifugal dissidents, who see themselves as seeking a different and more valid mode of worship. Following our definition, the former are sects and the latter are cults.

The distinction is exemplified by two groups whose roots lie in Judaism. The Lubavitch Hassidic group, a sect that traces its origins back two centuries, can claim legitimacy by all the criteria of classical Judaism. It has been reaching out to troubled young

Jews and, with a carefully designed program, has tried to engage and hold them. In their emphasis on ecstatic modes of worship, on archaic attire, and on dynastic community organization, the Hassidim set themselves apart from other orthodox Jews. But their deviations are inward, toward traditional forms, rather than outward, toward the alien. By the definition we suggest, this centripetal group would be called a sect rather than a cult.

Almost contemporaneously with the appearance of Hassidism in Eastern Europe, there appeared a small but active group led by a charismatic adventurer, Jacob Frank. He was able to recruit some of the residue of a failed messianic movement led by Sabbatai Zevi a century before. This new group turned away from traditional Judaism by embracing orgiastic sexuality as a mode of worship and ultimately accepting baptism into the Catholic Church. They also plotted against the Jews with their enemies, supporting accusations of blood libel. By the early nineteenth century, the group had largely dissolved. In terms of the definition we suggest, this centrifugal group would be called a cult.

While the distinction between cult and sect is important when studying the philosophy or rationale of a given group, cults and sects tend to be similar in structure and organization. Thus there is some justification for considering them together when describing these latter aspects.

References

Appel W: Cults in America: Programmed for Paradise. New York, Holt, Rinehart, and Winston, 1983

Cushman P: The Politics of Vulnerability. Psychohistory Review 12(4):5–17, 1984

Jewish Community Council of Philadelphia: The Challenge of the Cults, 1978

Melton JG: Encyclopedic Handbook of Cults in America. New York, Garland Publishing Co, 1984

Chapter 2

Is Psychiatry Relevant?

Different disciplines will provide different perspectives from which to study cults. Theologians have characterized religious groups in terms of the form of their beliefs, as gnostic, millenarian, messianic, heretical, liturgical, mystical, evangelical, or charismatic. Sociologists describe the cult's relation to society in such terms as deviance, marginality, and radicalism. Social psychologists study leadership styles and patterns of relationship within the group. Anthropologists look for indicators of tribal or ethnic cohesiveness, gender role differentiation, and collectively held mythical conceptions.

Psychiatrists too have a special approach to contribute to the study of cults. We are in a unique position to understand the personalities, needs, and motivations of the individuals who lead cults and of those who constitute their membership. We are in possession of a system for categorizing behaviors, thoughts, and affects in terms of their defensive and adaptive purposes. We can discriminate between unusual behaviors that serve a developmental end and those behaviors that are clearly pathological under any circumstances.

In his article "The Politics of Vulnerability: Youth in Religious Cults" Philip Cushman (1984) wrote about the aggressive recruitment methods of many cults and the ready availability of young people with shaky identities who are likely to be victims of these methods. He identifies the propensity of cults to abuse power by exploiting the powerless. These are the psychologically frail young persons, often naive in the ways of the world, prone to poorly reflected idealism, who are at the time of recruitment in a state of developmental transition, in need of friendship, authoritative guidance, and a sense of meaning. Cushman thus explains psychiatry's legitimate concern with cults: there is a population that is potentially at the mercy of religious entrepreneurs who have low regard for individuality, self-determination, and personal growth.

Cushman's article contains many first-hand accounts of prevailing recruitment and induction techniques aimed at fostering a symbiosis between leaders and members; this symbiosis interrupts the individuation process that psychiatrists believe is necessary and normal. Such frontal attacks upon the self by cults aiming at self-transcendence threaten the mental health of the unprepared who suffer from incomplete differentiation between themselves and others, as described by Engler (1983). In such instances, cults are symptom reinforcing rather than symptom relieving, so that the "cure" may be worse than the ailment.

Another practice of some cults is an insistence that inductees not only disown their original religion but also distance themselves from their families. This process is often accomplished in the context of seductive "love bombing" by proselytizers who—for the time being—overplay the role of "good parent." By inducing a cognitive and emotional regression, they "capture" the recruit. Feelings of alienation from the family of origin are manipulated so as to encourage discord and effect estrangement. Instead of healing family rifts or fostering the overdue process of separation-individuation, this kind of cult sows discord, encourages emotional constriction, and interferes with personal growth.

Some cult leaders have become known as pious frauds who accumulate immense personal wealth and claim a quasi-divine status that legitimatizes their desire for absolute control over their followers. This view may not be perceived by the group or it may be condoned or lauded. As psychiatrists we may speculate that those followers who idealize this behavior share the leader's penchant for deviousness, hypocrisy, and self-deception. These characteristics are all variants of the basic primitive defense mechanism of denial and permit the wide scale dissembling and cheating in the name of higher religious aims that is often observed. In this case, fraudulent leadership reinforces or worsens the developmental arrest and poor reality testing that made cult followers easy targets for proselytizers in the first place (Pruyser 1977, 1978).

In undertaking any assessment of cults, psychiatrists must be aware of elements unique to their own personal and professional experience, which might influence their perspective and interfere with objectivity. Among these experiences is a history of previous encounters with neurotic and psychotic distortions of religious thought. All varieties of religion have proven to be highly vulnerable to idiosyncratic, sometimes psychotic distortions (GAP Report 67, 1968). The psychiatrist's attitudes may be selectively influenced by those relatively few cult members or ex-members and their relatives who have appealed to them for help. Few psychiatrists participate in the ongoing life of cults, and most cult members avoid psychiatrists. Finally, self-scrutiny may make the psychiatrist aware of competitive feelings toward cults, evoked by the latter's use of "pop" psychology and therapeutic techniques. This rivalry has been described by Kilbourne and Richardson (1984).

References

Appel W: Cults in America: Programmed for Paradise. New York, Holt, Rinehart, and Winston, 1983

Cushman P: The politics of vulnerability. Psychohistory Review 12(4):5–17, 1984

Engler JH: Vicissitudes of the self according to psychoanalysis and Buddhism: a spectrum model of object relations development. Psychoanalysis and Contemporary Thought 6(1):29–72, 1983

Group for the Advancement of Psychiatry: The Psychic Function of Religion in Mental Illness and Health, formulated by the Committee on Psychiatry and Religion, 1968

Kaslow F, Sussman MB (eds): Cults and the Family. New York, Haworth Press (Marriage and Family Review, Vol 4, No 3/4), 1982

Kilbourne B, Richardson JT: Psychotherapy and New Religions in a Pluralistic Society. American Psychologist 3:237–251, 1984

Pruyser PW: The Seamy Side of Current Religious Beliefs. Bulletin of the Menninger Clinic 41:329–348, 1977

Chapter 3

Cults in the United States

This brief look at the development of cults in the United States aims to illustrate the social and cultural milieu in which cults are likely to arise. Similar groups are to be found throughout the Western world. Personal and psychological factors will be discussed later.

The Enlightenment of the eighteenth century was an era of optimistic belief that all knowledge could be attained through rational thought. Freemasonry, a fraternal organization based, among other things, on the ideal of religious toleration, and Deism, a system of thought which rejected organized religion, were popular among intellectuals, including the founding fathers. In their extroverted, rational orientation, these systems could in no way be considered cultlike.

Some cults arose during the nineteenth-century religious revival. The most prominent was The Church of Jesus Christ of the Latter Day Saints—the Mormons. It was founded in New York in the 1820s by Joseph Smith after he experienced religious revelations. The group moved to various sites across the country, finally settling in Utah, on the American frontier, in 1847. Smith, assassinated in Illinois, was replaced by Brigham Young. Perhaps the relative freedom of frontier society was a permissive factor in the group's growth and organization. The group flourished and is now accepted as a mainstream religion.

The Communalists lived according to the beliefs of their leader, John Humphrey Noyes. He claimed that the age of the New Zion had come and, basing his teaching on a passage in the book of St. Matthew 22:30 ("For in the resurrection they neither marry nor are given in marriage, but are as the angels of God in heaven"), dictated that followers live in communally owned property in which members did not have exclusive relationships.

Westward expansion made little provision for the Indian way of life. Forced by the government to live in reservations, their religious beliefs challenged by missionaries, and a principal food source—the buffalo—destroyed, Indians saw their culture devastated. Two major religious movements arose in response: The Ghost Dance and the Native American Church.

The Ghost Dance was a millennial movement founded in 1889 by a Northern Paiute named Wovoka. It was believed that "The Dance would hasten the coming of the renewed earth, where the living would be reunited with the dead, game would be plentiful, and the White Man would no longer be dominant over the Indian" (Halperin 1983). The movement died out, weakened by the Wounded Knee massacre in 1890 and the passing of the spring of 1891, the date set for millennial redemption.

The Native American Church, based on the ritual use of peyote, began among the Kiowa, Comanche, and Navajo. Peyote ingestion was used as a method of gaining insight to help in dealing with problems of everyday living, and their common religious practice served to unite the various tribes.

Similar circumstances contributed to cult formation in the Hawaiian Islands. With settlement by foreigners, the life of the native population was tragically altered. Diseases to which they had no immunity reduced the population from 300,000 in 1778 to 28,000 by the end of the nineteenth century. The Congregational Church replaced the old religious system, and descendants of the missionaries eventually dominated the business community. The missionaries altered the Hawaiian language when they put it into print. The overthrow of the monarchy gave the coup de grace to the Hawaiian attempt to regain autonomy.

Beginning in the 1850s the Hawaiian cult of Kaona attempted to bring back a way of life that was fast disappearing. Joseph Kaona, a native who had been a member of the Hawaiian House of Representatives and a district magistrate, studied the millennial teachings of the Millerites, who envisioned the end of the world and the second coming. Kaona became convinced that he was God and had visions. "Kaona was one of a long line of native prophets in the Pacific who came to realize that time was running out for their people, and whose revelations made it clear that nothing but a universal convulsion could bring back a world without white men" (Daws 1969). By 1868 Kaona had acquired a following of a few hundred who gave up their belongings, dressed in white robes, and settled on land they called "Lehuula" (red ashes). There they chanted, danced, and prayed, awaiting the end of the world. When the owner of the land on which they had settled attempted to regain it by force, the Kaonites killed the sheriff who led the posse and were arrested. Kaona was sent to prison and the cult disbanded.

Mary Baker Eddy established Christian Science in 1875 following the publication of her book, *Science and Health*. Eddy believed that God ruled the material world through a system of laws, and that illness, like sin, could be overcome by a proper mental attitude. This attempted rebuttal to scientific doctrine and Protestant ideals "provided some sort of resolution for the key anxieties of the era" (Albanese 1981).

The founder of the Shakers (formally called the United Society of Believers in Christ's Second Appearing), Mother Ann Lee, was regarded by her followers as Christ returned in the second coming. The popular name of the group was derived from its ritual dance, a trembling brought about by intense religious fervor. Believing that God possessed both male and female natures, and that sex was evil, the group lived communally and practiced celibacy.

Two movements that developed among American Blacks can be seen as a response to their disadvantaged position in society. Father Divine's Peace Mission was a syncretistic blend of Pentecostal faith, positive thinking, and secular pragmatism. It became an emotional support system for hundreds of American Blacks who were struggling in the process of urbanization. In return for submission to the group, which regarded Divine as the personification of God, members received food, clothing, and housing at minimal cost. In addition, the Mission supported civil rights and welfare for the poor.

The Black Jews began in Harlem around 1919. Claiming to be descendants of Ethiopian Jews, the Falashas, they rejected the term "Negro" and regarded Christianity as foreign. They claimed Hebrew as their original sacred tongue and observed Jewish dietary laws. Their religious services were somber and restrained, in contrast to those of the Southern Baptists and Pentecostals with whom they had been affiliated before coming North. George Simpson, a historian, speculated that "they invented a history, a culture, and a religion in an attempt to escape the stigma of being black and from being rejected by whites" (Simpson 1978).

The period between the two World Wars did not see a proliferation of cults, perhaps because the grim economic realities of the time affected individuals of all ages and classes and united families in a common response. By contrast, the conflict surrounding the

Vietnam War resulted in demoralization and alienation, particularly among the nation's youth, and gave rise to a number of new social organizations, including hippies, the drug culture, and encounter groups, as well as a spate of new cults.

Modern communications technology enabled those American youth searching for inspiration outside of their immediate culture to turn to the religions of India and Japan. Many ideas and practices of orthodox Eastern religious tradition were imported piecemeal and integrated into the beliefs of new religions and quasi-religious organizations were formed in the 1960s and subsequently.

Transcendental Meditation (TM), originally propounded by the Indian guru Maharishi Mahesh Yogi to adherents organized as a cult, is a technique whereby a "mantra" is chanted in order to achieve a state of religious "transcendence". Subsequently TM has been exported from the cult environment and taught in formal courses to almost a million Americans, most of whom use it in a nonreligious context to achieve physical and mental relaxation.

The Divine Light Mission, founded by Sri Hans Ji Maharaj in 1960, employed Yoga exercises to achieve spiritual enlightenment. Ji Maharaj died a year after the Mission's founding and was succeeded by his eight-year-old son, Maharaj Ji. Membership dropped after the latter was called back to India by his mother who complained that he was too hedonistic.

The Church of Scientology was founded around its Leader, L. Ron Hubbard. Hubbard became widely known through his book, *Dianetics*. Scientology combines Eastern and Western beliefs and teaches that self-knowledge will enable followers to express "the good innate within the self."

The International Society of Krishna Consciousness, or ISKON (Hare Krishnas), founded by A.C. Bhaktivendanta Swami Prabhupada, appeared on the scene in 1965. Still an active group, devotees live an ascetic life-style that includes ritual bathing, marking of the body with clay, worship to statues of deities, and chanting. Long hours are devoted to study of the Bhagavad Gita, and to proselytizing.

Zen Buddhism and Nichiren Shoshu, Buddhist sects with a long religious tradition in Japan, have both been imported intact to the United States where their practice and organization are more cultlike. The latter has acquired a huge following and is permeating mainstream American life through a sophisticated, well-financed campaign directed at the nation's public elementary schools.

The 1978 mass suicide and murder of The People's Temple in Jonestown, Guyana, epitomized the horror that could result from cult participation. Pathological loss of self-will enabled many of Jones's followers to kill themselves or others with little or no resistance. This incident led to increased interest in the psychology of cult leaders and their followers.

This sketch of a few of the innumerable cults that have proliferated in the United States illustrates how varied cults have been in practice, credo, and durability. Some cults died out within a few years of their founding, while others have endured, and still others, such as the Mormons and the Christian Scientists, have been incorporated into the religious mainstream. Some ideas about what contributes to the popularity and durability of a cult will be discussed in a subsequent chapter.

References

Albanese C: American Religions and Religion. Belmont, CA, Wadsworth Publishing, 1981

Bainbridge W, Stark R: Cult formation: three compatible models. Sociological Analysis 40(4):283, 1979

Billias G, Grob G: American History. New York, Free Press, 1971

Clausen H: Masons Who Helped Shape the Nation. San Diego, CA, Neyensch Printers, 1976

Cornault F: Les Frances des Sectes. Paris, Tchou, 1978

Daws G: Shoal of Time. New York, NY, Macmillan Company, 1969

Downey W: Admitted to the Mysteries. New York, Exposition Press, 1970

Ellwood R: Religious and Spiritual Groups in Modern America, Englewood Cliffs, NJ, Prentice-Hall, 1973

Enroth R: Youth, Brainwashing, and the Extremist Cults. Grand Rapids, MI, Zondervan Corp, 1977

Galanter M: Charismatic religious sects and psychiatry. American Journal of Psychiatry 139:1539–1548, 1982

Gaustad E (ed): A Documentary History of Religion in America, Vol II. Grand Rapids, MI, William Eerdman Publishing Co, 1982

Halperin A (ed): Psychodynamic Perspectives of Religion, Sect, and Cult. New York, John Wright Publishing Co, 1983

Hoffer E: The True Believer: Thoughts on the Nature of Mass Movements. New York, New American Library, 1951

Jones B: Freemason's Book of the Royal Arch. London, George C. Harrup & Co. 1965

Kaplan H, Sadock B (eds): Comprehensive Textbook of Psychiatry V. Baltimore, MD, Williams & Wilkins, 1990

Kaslow F, Sussman M (eds): Cults and the Family. New York, Haworth Press, 1982

Kodama M: Kaona Insurrection of 1868: Its Background and Analysis. Unpublished Undergraduate Paper. University of Hawaii Library, 1968

Koch A: Cults and Mental Health: Clinical Conclusions. Canadian Journal of Psychiatry 26:534–539, 1981

Ling T: A History of Religion East and West. London, Macmillan Press, 1979

Morais H: Deism in 18th Century America. New York, Columbia Press, 1934

McDermott JF Jr, et al (eds): People and Cultures. Honolulu, HI, University Press of Hawaii, 1980

Melton JG, Moore R: The Cult Experience. New York, Pilgrim Press, 1982

Miller E: Authoritarianism: The American Cults and Their Intellectual Antecedents. University of Hawaii Library, 1979

Mosely J: A Cultural History of Religion in America. Connecticut, Greenwood Press, 1981

Pavlos A: The Cult Experience. Connecticut, Greenwood Press, 1982

Prabhupada AC: Bhaktivedanta, Bhagavad Gita As It Is. New York, The Bhaktivedanta Book Trust, 1973

Ross M: Clinical Profiles of Hari Krishna Devotees. American Journal of Psychiatry 140:416–429, 1983

Simpson G: Black Religions in the New World. New York, Columbia University Press, 1978

The Holy Bible, King James Version. New York, Abradale Press

Chapter 4

Cult Leaders

In 1972, a 35-year-old American calling himself Baba returned from an Indian ashram and began daily sittings on a park bench in New York City. He had never experienced a happy family life: His father killed his mother and then committed suicide when Baba was 21, and Baba left his own wife and children when he was 30.

During the next four years he acquired about 30 followers who, interestingly enough, called themselves "The Family" (Deutsch 1975). Vegetarian meals were prepared in a disciple's nearby apartment, and Baba and most of the others slept on an adjoining rooftop. Baba spoke only in sign language, translated to outsiders by his first disciple, Sid. During the day Baba held forth on religious themes to passersby.

About five months after Baba began his sittings, The Family purchased an old bus and moved to a hilltop in a nearby state. There, some 100 followers formed a farm commune. No vows were taken, and people came and went as they wished. Baba's central teaching was the necessity of letting go of attachments to ambition, sex, possessions, and guilt.

Baba's behavior became increasingly bizarre, sadistic, and domineering. He often struck his disciples and was sexually abusive with some of the women. By 1975 he had deteriorated to the point where his sign language was unintelligible even to his closest followers, and he was grimacing constantly. He saw his former Indian teacher as the devil incarnate and wanted no more followers. The commune disbanded, and Baba's fate is unknown.

In 1965, a 67-year-old retired pharmaceutical executive from India, A.C. Bhaktivendanta Swami Prabhupada, came to New York City with six dollars in his pocket and founded the Interna-

17

tional Society of Krishna Consciousness (ISKON). In India Prabhupada had been a follower of a Krishna sect and had edited its "Back to Godhead" magazine. At age 58 he forsook all ties to his wife, five children, and job and became a Hindu monk. Nine years later he came to New York to begin his teaching.

Beginning in a storefront mission in the lower East Side, he offered free vegetarian meals while preaching his message of worship of the Lord Krishna as the personal manifestation of the Godhead, using as his text the Indian spiritual classic the Bhagavad Gita. His early followers were mostly youths from the hippie culture.

ISKON, commonly known as the Hare Krishnas, grew rapidly, aided by the publicity it received by attracting the poet Alan Ginsberg, Beatle George Harrison, and the rock group The Grateful Dead. The group has become familiar to the public through its orange-robed, shaven headed devotees intoning their Hare Krishna chant on urban streets and requesting donations in return for a flower. Today the movement seems well established, having survived Swami Prabhupada's death in 1977. One contribution to its success was the founder's foresight in appointing governing commissioners to oversee the movement before he died. There are now about 40 temples in Europe, Australia, and New Zealand.

These examples, both derived from the Indian religious scene, illustrate two contrasting outcomes of a cult. In the first, Baba's psychotic disorganization caused the cult to be abandoned. In the second, Prabhupada presided over the group's growth until his death and wisely made plans for the group beyond his own survival. Many factors determine if a cult will flourish, but the figure of the leader is a major factor (Deutsch 1980).

The Figure of the Leader

Study of the cult leader has been rather neglected, most of the attention being focused on the followers. The typical cult leader is by nature not likely to offer himself or herself as a subject for evaluation by a mental health professional. Descriptions made available by the cults themselves present their leaders in a favorable, larger-than-life portrait that masks their actual personalities. Nonetheless, it is possible to make inferences from these portraits about the cult leader's ideal self-image. Certain aspects are typically encountered and contribute to the mythology prevailing among his followers. These include: The Hero, The Outsider, The Narcissist, The Charismatic Figure, and The Entrepreneur. Any particular leader can manifest more than one of these aspects in combination. Because most leaders among the cults we have studied are men, the male pronoun is used throughout the paragraphs that follow.

The Hero. He is portrayed in Joseph Campbell's *The Hero With a Thousand Faces* (Campbell 1968). Typically the Hero is born in relative obscurity, during a time of danger or turmoil. Prophecies often herald his coming. Frequently he is said to have one divine parent and one human parent. He displays extraordinary capacities early in life: prodigious strength and extreme precocity involving wisdom or cleverness. His powers develop during a period of relative obscurity. An event then occurs in which the Hero recognized his uniqueness and the calling to a chosen mission. He may disregard this for a time but eventually embarks on a mission that will be attended by suffering and pitfalls.

The Outsider. The leader has generally been an outsider in relation to the mainstream. He feels alienated and opposed, he spends his life compensating. By acquiring an intensely loyal band of followers he creates a world in which he is the supreme insider. He takes an adversarial stance toward the outside world, regarding it as something to fear, avoid, manipulate, or "save." Hence the leader comes to see himself as the persecuted savior.

The Narcissist. "By taking on the identity of master [the leader] acquires an identity that carries with it the numinosity of the Self in its most undiluted concrete form" (Satinover 1980). The leader, and to a much lesser extent his disciples, live in the infant's narcissistic world of fantasies of grandeur and power, modified as little as possible by limitations and frustration. Whatever difficulties are encountered within the cult and outside are seen by the leader as flaws in an imperfect and unenlightened humanity, as goading obstacles to be overcome on the way to perfection. Typically, leaders leave their nuclear families to pursue their calling, and the external world is regarded as subservient to the mission.

The Charismatic Figure. Max Weber defines charisma as "a certain quality of an individual personality by virtue of which he is set apart from ordinary men and treated as endowed with supernatural, superhuman, or at least specifically exceptional qualities or properties" (Weber, original 1922, translated 1947). The cult and the leader desperately need each other. The leader must be the bearer for all the idealizations and projections attributed to him by his followers. He must successfully project these attributes. To do this his belief in his own uniqueness and calling and his ability to convince others of this are indispensable. As we shall see, the followers are in dire need of an anointed figure.

The Entrepreneur. If the cult is to expand beyond a small unit, the leader must be in part an entrepreneur. A growing cult needs a marketing aspect to carry on its quest for new recruits and money. Almost all leaders of successful large cults are accomplished entrepreneurs. Trusted followers may assist in this task as the organization becomes increasingly complex.

Cults whose leaders lack this combination of traits will probably fail to grow beyond a small band that depends on personal contact between leader and disciple. This kind of cult will not survive the loss of its leader.

The Reverend Sun Myung Moon

As an illustration, let us look in some detail at the career of one of the most successful leaders of contemporary "new religions"—The Reverend Sun Myung Moon (Bromley and Shupe 1979). His Holy Spirit Association for the Unification of World Christianity (more succinctly, the Unification Church) has become a stable and, no doubt, an enduring presence. In the past fifteen years it has been the nidus of intense conflict between its members and irate parents and deprogrammers. While the target of anti-cultists' barrages, its rights have been defended by the American Civil Liberties Union and the National Council of Churches. The group in the United States has grown from about 20 full-time members in 1960 to 6000 in 1980. The current holdings of the Unification Church in this country are said to be valued at about $200 million.

The Reverend Moon was born in northern Korea in 1920 during the harsh Japanese occupation. He was the fifth of eight children in a rural family. When Moon was ten years old, the family joined a Presbyterian church with Pentecostal practices. As a child, it is reported, he wept for the sorrows of Jesus, experienced oneness with nature, and protested with tears and tantrums any mistreatment of children by adults.

Moon has said that when he was age 16, Jesus appeared to him during his prayers, confessed that his own work was incomplete, and said that God had chosen Moon to complete the mission of establishing His kingdom on earth. During the next nine years, Moon made an intense search for religious truth. In this search he encountered "cosmic evil" and communicated with Jesus, Moses, and Buddha.

Moon had a traditional Chinese education in his village and attended high school in Seoul. In 1941 he matriculated in electrical engineering in Japan, returning to Korea two years later to carry on in this occupation. Accused of supporting Korean independence, he was imprisoned by the Japanese for four months in the following year.

It was then that he felt the need to choose among being an engineer, a political activist, or a religious leader. In 1945, at the age of 25, he decided on the last course. The following year it was revealed to him that he was to start a ministry in the north Korean city of Pyong-Yang. Leaving his wife and two-month-old child, he established an independent church there. Moon was opposed by both the ruling Communists (the Japanese had been defeated by this time) and the orthodox Christians, and he was twice jailed and tortured. When he was released from a labor camp by United Nations forces in 1950 he set off with two faithful companions, one of whom had a broken leg, for Pusan, 600 miles to the south. They arrived by bicycle. He and his followers, whom he had instructed to meet him there, set up their church in a Pusan refugee camp. Moon supported himself through employment as a dockworker.

He established his church in Seoul in 1954, using its present name, and issued the first version of *The Divine Principle*. He was imprisoned again the following year, allegedly for fostering adultery and promiscuity within the church. The church itself has stated that it was for an unsubstantiated charge of draft evasion. The charge was dropped and Moon was released after three months. Shortly after, the church was moved to Cheong Prabong, its present world headquarters.

Expansion of the Unification Church began in the late 1950s. The first missionary went to Japan in 1958, and Dr. Yung Don Kim went to the United States in 1959. She had been a professor of comparative religion in a Seoul university until she was expelled in 1955 because of her membership in the Unification Church. While a graduate student in Canada, she had had a series of mystical experiences. Others were also sent to the United States and Europe; at first the results were negligible. Several small groups remained relatively autonomous, and each took on the character of the local leader.

A systematic training program for new members in a communal setting was instituted in Japan with great success, though enemies called it brainwashing. It was subsequently transplanted to the United States. A commune was established in San Francisco in 1965.

Moon himself provided the major impetus for growth in the West. After making three world tours, he returned to the United

States in 1971 to announce that America was to play a more active role in the establishment of God's kingdom. He brought the disparate groups together, retrained and shuffled leaders, and encouraged members to spend more time on the streets raising money. Moon himself made numerous appearances in revival meetings in large cities.

With growth came increasing expenses. An eight-city tour, including a massive rally at Madison Square Garden, was reported to have cost a million dollars. Large-scale fund raising became a major enterprise. Teams began selling candles, peanuts, and flowers and requesting donations. Due to the success of this program the church has acquired considerable property, both for its own use and for commercial purposes.

Through all this growth the church retained a familial organization. Moon had dissolved his first marriage because his wife disapproved of his religious activity, but he married again in 1960. He and his second wife were looked upon as the spiritual parents of the members. He maintained close supervision over the union of couples and instituted the practice of mass weddings for movement members. The largest of these occurred in the United States in 1975 when Moon officiated at the union of 1800 couples. This emphasis on marriage has doubtless been made to establish more stable relations within the group. Further, the church has consistently encouraged large families and discouraged birth control and abortion, partly, at least, to ensure growth of the movement.

Moon has formed several subsidiary groups that help tie the church to different segments of society. These groups include the International Cultural Foundation, the annual International Conference on the Unity of Sciences, the Professors' World Peace Academy, and The Confederation for the Unification of the Societies of the Americas (CAUSA). The last is chiefly concerned with combating communism in Latin America. The church also owns numerous newspapers both here and abroad, including *The Washington Times* and its weekly newsmagazine, *Insight*.

In 1984 Moon was convicted of income tax evasion in the United States, fined $25,000, and sentenced to prison for 18 months. With time off for good behavior, he served 13 months and was released in August 1985. Numerous clergy came to his defense, asserting that this prosecution constituted federal intrusion into a religious matter and did not fall within the purview of the court.

The belief system of the Unification Church, as outlined in *The Divine Principle*, is a blend of Western Christianity and Asian tradition. It asserts that mankind is alienated from its true parent,

God, because of Eve's fornication with the archangel Lucifer in Eden and the subsequent Fall. Restoration of man's proper relation to God requires the coming of the Messiah. The first Messiah, Jesus, almost succeeded in paying the necessary indemnity, but his early death prevented him from marrying and establishing the model God-centered family. For this reason, Jesus succeeded in establishing spiritual salvation but failed to establish physical salvation. The second Messiah will achieve the latter by creating a prototypical family. The Divine Principle claims that this second Messiah was to be born around 1920 in Korea but does not mention Moon's name. Moon himself has evaded this issue, although he has referred to himself in a messianic way. Most members believe that Moon is the Messiah.

Moon clearly qualifies as a successful leader. The accounts of his life may not be accurate, but they portray the man as he and his followers wish him to be seen. He has all the typical features of the cult leader that were described earlier.

Moon's life, as depicted for his followers, follows Campbell's prototype of The Hero. While he has a human father, he also has a divine one, for God has chosen him as a second son—a Messiah. In childhood, his differences set him apart from others: intolerance of aggression toward children, a sense of identity with the cosmos, and religious emotionalism. In adolescence he encountered Jesus and experienced his first summon to become the new Messiah. Characteristic of the heroic quest, he has survived persecution, trial, and imprisonment, and he has prospered.

As an intensely religious child, Moon was The Outsider in his own family. He continued as an outsider when he was a political activist against the Japanese invader, and he was an outsider in attempting to form a cult. As the founder and leader of a cult, he found a perfect solution, for he created a world in which he was the supreme Insider.

As one who shows the way to the second Messiah, if not considering himself the Messiah, Moon manifests the grandiosity of the Narcissist. Certainly, he has been a Charismatic Figure to his followers, and equally, he has been a highly successful Entrepreneur. Continuity is a problem faced by all cults, and it is likely that the Unification Church will continue for a long time. The longevity of a cult and its ultimate recognition as an accepted religion are determined in fair measure by the entrepreneurial talents of the leader and his successors.

References

Bromley DG, Shupe AD: "Moonies" in America. Beverly Hills, CA, Sage Publications, 1979

Deutsch A: Observations on a Sidewalk Ashram. Archives of General Psychiatry 32:165–175, 1975

Deutsch A: Tenacity of attachment to a cult leader: a psychiatric perspective. American Journal of Psychiatry 137:1569–1573, 1980

Campbell J: The Hero With a Thousand Faces. Princeton, NJ, Princeton University Press, 1968

Satinover J: Puer Aeternus: the narcissistic relation to the self. Quadrant 13:75–108, 1980

Weber M: The Theory of Social and Economic Organization. Glencoe, NY, Free Press, 1947, p 358

Chapter 5

Cult Followers

While there is no doubt that cults and cult membership have proliferated during the past two decades, surveys differ widely in their estimates of the actual numbers involved. Of course, estimates will depend on one's definition or conception of a cult and whether the count is restricted to fully participating members. Statistics provided by the cults themselves are often at variance with the results of surveys made by outsiders.

Conway and Siegelman (1978) estimated about 3 million cult members, past and present, in the United States. This is a far cry from Gallup Poll projections (1978) that 8.5 million teenagers were involved in one of the "new religions," and that the number had risen to more than 13 million in 1981—over 50% of all teenagers in the country. Gallup's figures apparently represent the extent of interest in the cults, rather than actual involvement. Full-time involvement in the better known cults turns out to be but a small fraction of the total membership in Gallup's sense. ISKON has claimed 5000 full-time members, in contrast to Gallup's figure of 375,000. Similarly, the Unification Church claimed a membership of 37,000, contrasting with Gallup's figure of 400,000.

Cult membership does not reflect a cross-section of the population (Galanter 1979). Most members are not from the underprivileged classes but are middle class, young, white, single, and relatively well educated. Males outnumber females by about two to one. In a survey of 119 newly affiliated members of the Divine Light Mission, Galanter found that 97% were white, 82% single, and 73% in their twenties. Seventy-six percent of the members and one or both parents of 71% had attended college. Among members of the Unification Church, 89% were white, 91% single, and their mean age was 24.7 years. Most came from intact families and were partially or wholly dependent on their parents for support at the time they joined the church.

Who Joins

In an effort to characterize those who enter cults, a number of variables have been considered: social and cultural factors, family and religious background, personality characteristics, and developmental difficulties. All of the factors that predispose individuals to join cults may also contribute to psychopathology. In fact, many individuals who join cults show evidence of previous psychopathology, though estimates differ as to its nature and degree of severity. The fact that cults appeal to late adolescents and young adults directs our attention to developmental concerns in these age groups.

Social and Cultural Factors

The Vietnam War, the nuclear arms race, and the resultant fear of nuclear disaster are commonly considered to have undermined established institutions and spawned the counterculture of the late 1960s and 1970s. In addition, many feel that the burgeoning of technology and bureaucracy has been dehumanizing and has led to fear of loss of individualism. There is no generally accepted proof for either of these hypotheses.

The counterculture offered new political, social, sexual, and religious options. These options were adopted by many young adults who felt disappointed by the established social order. For others, the new freedom was frightening. The cults were particularly attractive to this latter group; many joined after becoming disillusioned or frightened by their experiences with drugs, sex, or other aspects of the counterculture. Cult membership permitted, even demanded, rebellion against conventional society while it provided an alternative source of structure, purpose, and support.

The Religious Factor

Definitive data regarding the religious upbringing of cult members are not available, but one thing seems certain: those from strong religious backgrounds are less likely to join cults than those without such backgrounds. Relatively few devotees come from observant Catholic or Orthodox Jewish families, while a disproportionately large number are Jews from liberal, nonobservant families. It should be borne in mind that the religious attitudes of young people are often determined by the nature of their relationships to their parents. Those who feel rebellious in the context of a structured religious atmosphere will be unlikely to feel attracted to the dogmatic, structured life-style of the cults. On the other hand, cults have appealed to many who saw their less observant families as insincere in their beliefs.

Family Background

Our clinical experience suggests that difficulties in achieving normal adult separation from family is a prime motivation for joining a cult. Most cult members come from intact, close-knit, middle-class, achievement-oriented families. For them, the cult may enable a counter-dependent rebellion against family by providing a substitute group with similar dynamic characteristics. We wondered whether some families are particularly "cultogenic."

It seems clear that there is no one personality pattern or central conflict that is specific to those who chose to join cults. However, sociologists and psychologists have enumerated the following several family characteristics that may so predispose children: 1) Authoritarian, protective parents who fail to prepare children for the adult task of decision making. A child from such a background may need to seek out a group in which all decisions are made by others. 2) Overly permissive parents who do not provide a consistent system of values and expectations. Children from these homes may fail to internalize an adequate set of ideals on which to base adult identity. The charismatic nature of the cult leader may appear particularly attractive to them. 3) Families that demand more than the child can achieve. Their children may find comfort in the fact that cults do not demand achievement and may even discourage it. 4) Families that seem sound and lack overt conflict but are somehow without warmth. Their children may find the initial "love bombing" especially seductive. 5) Parents who fail to give their children a sense of being valued as adults. In this case, children may not be motivated to mature into psychological adulthood. As cult members they can remain children indefinitely, without the shame of having to remain with their families as dependents who "couldn't make it."

Hardat Sukhdeo (1981), a psychiatrist who has worked with many cult members, has published his own description of the families he typically encounters: They are small and inward-looking, centered around the nuclear family. The father is often passive and the mother is often domineering. The parents tend to be children of first- or second-generation immigrants, torn between the values of their own parents and the wish to assimilate American ideals. They are generally determined to win for their children the material comforts, education, and financial security that they did not themselves have. Many of these parents have paid the price that a conflict of values often extracts—a disinclination to trust their own feelings and an inability to reveal them in communication with others.

The Cult Member: A Composite Picture

The white, middle-class, idealistic young people who form the majority in most contemporary cults are often lonely, depressed, and fearful of an uncertain future. They tend to be dependent. They have strong needs for affection. Unable to provide for their own emotional sustenance, they need external sources for a feeling of self-worth, a sense of belonging, and a reason for living. They feel resentful and are often openly hostile toward society at large; it has disappointed them and does not value them. The freedoms as well as the demands of young adulthood, eagerly awaited by many, may be overwhelming for them.

When questioned, members and ex-members give specific reasons for having become involved in cults. Among the more frequent responses are: feelings of loneliness and loss following separation from their families; setbacks in their emotional lives, such as disappointments in friends and love relationships; alienation from their environment, which they felt had failed to provide them with rules or direction; the feeling that they were drifting and that life had no meaning; a need for idealism and spirituality; and pressure from a friend or lover who was in the cult.

The motivation for joining cults may arise from the developmental challenges of late adolescence. Most basic is the need to assume an adult identity. It is our feeling that cult membership is a maladaptive way to achieve this in young people for whom the task is especially problematic. Many behaviors and relationships observed in cult members can be understood as attempts to solve the difficulties posed by the demands of adulthood.

The most pervasive of these behaviors, the persistence of strong dependency needs, can manifest as a wish to be cared for, or defensively, as rebelliousness. The disinclination to make choices and take responsibility for one's own life contributes to a desire to remain within the well-defined confines of a group where all decisions are made for members and the daily repetitive routine offers predictability and security.

Psychological testing of cult members is reported to confirm the presence of dependent traits, and frequently shows them to be associated with addictive features, that is, a need for external sources of gratification (Spero 1982). This need may explain the prevalence of problems with sexual and social relationships noted in many cult members. Dependence may also explain the high incidence of drug abuse among followers prior to joining the cult. It may be said that joining a cult is exchanging one addiction for another.

The type of cult chosen is important because they vary in the kind of behavioral restrictions imposed on individual members, the degree of thought control exercised by the leader, sexual practices, and the extent of captivity any member may experience. Individuals who require strong external controls over aggressive or sexual impulses will be attracted to ascetic cults that demand abstinence. Cults with more open living arrangements will appeal to those who can tolerate greater flexibility in relationships. Sexually permissive cults may help overcome conflicts associated with guilt over adult sexuality.

In addition to independence, productive adult life demands a degree of optimism and self-confidence. These qualities are lacking in cult members, who tend to suffer from poor self-esteem and an inclination to self-doubt. These latter traits, originating in childhood, are reinforced by a recent history of failure in school or in other activities. Low self-esteem is often accompanied by an intolerance for ambiguity; the quest for certainty leads to polarization of attitudes, disposition, and loyalties. Furthermore, poor self-confidence and faulty optimism may lead to rejection of conventional society and its values; but without society's ideals to aspire to, the young person is left without any direction or restraints, and can easily become confused and overwhelmed. The cult and the cult leader offer a ready solution. As one cult member put it, "Being told what to accept was a relief. You could give up the constant struggle."

A high proportion of cult members report that they had few close friends before joining and were unable to identify themselves with any place, institution, or occupation. The cult offers meaning, a sense of belonging, and even drama to an otherwise lonely existence. Here they feel they are doing good work; they may even save the world. They have become special. The revised self-image undoes the previous feeling of isolation and emptiness. A new and better society in which one plays an important role replaces the rejected group of origin.

Poor self-esteem and the resultant alienation will in turn cause an individual to become hostile, resenting those whom he or she feels unable to measure up to. Cult members justify these sentiments in a variety of ways. Some say they are reacting to a society that is corrupt and evil. Others blame their parents, whom they perceive to be hypocritical and inconsistent in their practices. The cult provides assistance with these hostile feelings by sanctioning their expression in defense of the cult's superior aims. This is sometimes accompanied by claims of love for every living creature. For those who fear the intensity of aggressive impulses, the rituals of cult life provide an external source of control that compensates for the lack of inner controls.

A significant number of cult members report episodes of disorientation or fragmentation accompanied by the sensation that their life is falling apart (Appel 1978). Erikson (1963) has referred to this state as "identity diffusion" and attributed it to "a combination of experiences which demand simultaneous commitment to physical intimacy, decisive occupational choice, energetic competition and psycho-social self-definition."

In essence, this fragmentation is a severe response to the demands of adulthood by those who cannot otherwise tolerate them. Apocalyptic cults may appeal particularly to young people in this state. The concept of world destruction resonates with their fears, while cult membership promises survival.

Incidence of Psychopathology

The characteristics we have described above may be manifestations of developmental problems, or they may be embedded in
more serious psychopathology. Reliable statistical data are not
available, as there is great variability among groups studied and
diagnostic criteria applied by investigators. Thus studies can rarely
be compared. Most agree that the majority of cult members suffer
from problems that antedate their commitment to the cult, but
estimates of the nature of the problems differ widely.

Willa Appel (1978) asserts that most cult members are essentially normal people who turn to cults at a moment of particular
difficulty in their lives. Psychologist Margaret Singer (1979) estimated that 75% of cult members are "basically normal." A study
based on 100 "rehabilitation" cases conducted by a deprogramming group, G. Kelly Associates, indicates that 68% (mostly ex-
members of the Unification Church) were "stable" individuals
who were experiencing "mild adolescent difficulties" at the time
of their conversion.

In contrast, psychiatrist John Clark (1978) has maintained
that some 60% of people in all stages of cult involvement, examined
by him personally, were "chronically disturbed." The other 40%
were found to be essentially normal, but susceptible to conversion
because of "crises of maturation" and pressure from an aggressive
proselytizer.

There is general agreement that seriously disturbed people
are a minority in cult populations. Truly psychotic individuals do
not make good converts or group members. Despite their initial
enthusiasm, they undergo a crisis sooner or later and revert to a
more autistic relationship to reality.

Spero (1982) has reported on the testing and therapy of 65
devotees. 35 were members of "mildly to seriously disturbed"
families; of these, 20 had histories of prior consultations with
psychiatrists or school psychologists. Psychological tests were
given to all 65 before, during, and after therapy, and revealed two
basic profiles: 1) significant constriction in cognitive processes with
a preference for stereotypy or 2) a manic denial of depressive
trends. The most important findings were problems in differenti-
ating between self and non-self and between inner and outer
reality. Twenty-four of the 65 manifested "borderline" phenomena. Three had frequent episodes of "slippage" or "floating" (that
is, attention disorders) during early months of treatment. Spero

also noted poor impulse control, narcissistic trends, a weakness of critical judgement, defensive "splitting" into good and bad selves, and an infantile quality in their orientation to reality and in their relations with others. While these findings are suggestive of psychosis or borderline states, Spero makes no firm diagnostic commitments nor does he indicate the incidence or severity of the pathology noted.

Although a control group of the same age and social status would be needed to draw more definitive conclusions, the overall impression gained from the literature is that most cult members show signs of personality or developmental disorders. No doubt, psychopathology of cult members is broadly spread among other diagnostic categories as well, not particularly different from the general population. The overall incidence of psychopathology is probably greater, but the extent of this difference is not known.

Who Leaves and Who Stays

Cults are reluctant to disclose information regarding duration of stay or rates of attrition. The fact that few cult members are over age 35 (less than 10% according to most surveys) suggests a high number of dropouts. Members are motivated to leave for a variety of reasons, often directly related to the reasons that motivated them to join in the first place. We can expect that differences will exist between those who leave voluntarily and those who are involuntarily abducted and deprogrammed.

As we have seen, many cult members become involved during a particular developmental stage, usually late adolescence, when they are confronted with problems they could not otherwise resolve, such as the need to separate from parents, to assume an identity as part of a group, and to feel special. As development continues, other things, such as the desire for marriage and parenthood, become important. Cult membership may no longer be necessary and may, in fact, pose a hindrance to these later achievements.

Continuing attachment to family and friends outside the cult constitutes a major motivation for leaving. The persistence of these ties gives rise to depression and guilt, and disillusionment with the cult may set in once the initial seduction is over. The monotony of the rigidly organized life upsets some members. For others, the sleep deprivation that results from a fully scheduled 18-hour day is intolerable.

A survey by Conway and Siegelman (1982) indicates that the majority of 400 cult members they studied experienced serious physical, mental, and emotional disturbances while in the cult. Physical complaints included extreme weight gain or loss, abnormal skin conditions, menstrual irregularities, and reduced facial hair growth among men. Emotional problems included guilt, fear, depression, suicidal impulses, and hostility, sometimes resulting in outbursts of violence. More than half experienced disturbances of perception, memory, and cognition. Whether or not these symptoms are manifestations of preexisting pathology, they indicate that the "cult option" has failed and can motivate members to leave.

Ungerleider and Wellisch (1979) conducted a study of 50 members or former members of religious cults who came to them to discuss the issue of deprogramming. They fell into four categories: The first were 22 "concerned members" who feared deprogramming. The second were 11 "returnees" who had been unsuccessfully deprogrammed. The third were 9 "non-returnees" who were successfully deprogrammed. The fourth were 8 "voluntary ex-members" who left the cults of their own volition.

Each subject was given a psychiatric examination and a battery of psychological tests. The two groups of cults members, the "concerned members" and the "returnees," displayed a greater degree of social and emotional alienation. They had significant difficulties with impulse control and superego deficits. For them, the cults served as external consciences. By encouraging repression and denial, they helped control hostility and drug intake.

Those who left voluntarily showed less need for a structured, predictable environment. While each of the other three groups were helped by the structured social situation of the cults, those who were successfully deprogrammed found this advantage counterbalanced by the feeling of being forced into a submissive role. Those who remained saw themselves as becoming more dominant within the cult. While some do rise in the hierarchy, the authors attributed the perception to impaired reality testing in most.

The two groups of people who remained in the cults manifested far more hostility toward their families than those who left. In some individuals, a brief period of hostility toward the cult leaders was quickly repressed and then projected onto people outside the cult.

Two factors are important in determining whether an individual will remain in a cult. One involves the cult's efficacy in solving the problems at hand. If membership results in diminished pain and frustration and closer relations, the tendency will be to remain. By the same token, a member will leave if he or she becomes further distressed. The second factor is the tenacity of the problems that motivated joining. Developmental problems and some personality disorders may be transient, so the need for the cult may diminish or disappear in time. When the problems are pervasive and fixed, as in borderline conditions, there will be a greater likelihood of remaining in the cult. Relatively healthy and capable members may also chose to stay in the cult if they achieve positions of power and influence.

References

Appel W: Cults in America. New York: Holt, Rinehart, and Winston, 1983

Clark JG Jr: The Manipulation of Madness. Unpublished paper presented in Hanover, Germany, 1978, p 12

Conway F, Siegelman J: Snapping. Philadelphia, PA, JB Lippincott, 1978

Information Disease: Have Cults Created a New Illness? Science Digest, January 1982, p 92

Erikson EH: Childhood and Society. New York, WW Norton, 1963

Galanter M, Rabkin R, Deutsch A: "The Moonies": A Psychological Study of Conversion and Membership in a Contemporary Religious Sect. American Journal of Psychiatry 136:165–169, 1979

Gallup G: Gallup Youth Survey. New York, NY, Associated Press, 1978, 1981

Singer M: Coming Out of the Cults. Psychology Today, January 1979, pp 72–82

Spero MH: Psychotherapeutic Procedure With Religious Cult Devotees. The Journal of Nervous and Mental Disease 170:332–344, 1982

Sukhdeo HAS: A Clinician's Reflections on Some of the Problems of the Jewish Family in Contemporary America. Unpublished pamphlet (see Appel 1983), 1983

Ungerleider JT, Wellisch DK: Coercive Persuasion (Brainwashing), Religious Cults and Deprogramming. American Journal of Psychiatry 136:279–282, 1979

Chapter 6

The Dead Sea Sects:
A Model for Modern Cults

A mong the obstacles that psychiatrists encounter in their efforts to understand the proliferation of cults in the Western
world of today, two problems can be partially overcome by taking
a similar institution from the ancient world as a model. First, the
personal feelings of sympathy or hostility that modern cults elicit
in the psychiatrist are less likely to be evoked. Second, the problem
of ascertaining what the group stands for is resolved in this case
by the availability of its actual scriptures.

Ancient scrolls found in caves near Qumran, south of Jericho,
and in ruins of a large building discovered nearby, permit the
reconstruction of the life of a collective community that set itself
up in the Judaean desert. Paleographic evidence, radioactive car-
bon techniques, and identification of coins establish that the community existed from some time during the second century B.C.
until the Jewish revolt against Rome that terminated in the fourth
decade of the second century A.D. The picture we can reconstruct
from these artifacts corresponds with descriptions provided by
classical historians of that period—including Josephus, Philo, and
Pliny—of a schismatic, sectarian group called the Essenes. Possibly
the identification is incorrect and the scriptures examined here
come from another similar group, but these concerns are immater-
ial for our purposes.

Although there were a number of desert groups whose
scriptures differ one from the other, the principal body of extant
writings maintains a fair degree of consistency. The Dead Sea
groups are ordinarily called sects, while those we are studying here

are ordinarily called cults. This complies with the distinction made in the section on definitions in that the Dead Sea groups practiced what they felt to be a purified form of the established religion, not a new one. But as we shall see, their organization was much like that of the cults we are studying.

The preserved documents on the Dead Sea groups will help us understand the psychodynamic expectations of the participants and give some idea of the relation of the group to the world around it. Perhaps the inferences from this study can be applied to current cultic phenomena.

Sect Structure and Rules of Behavior

The available chronicles show that the members of the group were subjected to strict discipline. The individual was required to defer to all group decisions. There was little room for individual initiative and none for idiosyncratic behavior. Not only were officers and leaders designated by group decision, but each member was assigned a specific status that was determined by the group on the basis of the individual's conduct. The discipline regulated the conduct required by differences in status, as well as matters of etiquette in dealings between each individual and his fellows, and between the individual and the community. Penalties and punishments, including expulsion from the community, are explained in detail.

Upon admission, all personal property was surrendered to the community. In return, the community accepted the obligation to provide for all the needs of its members.

Admission to the sect required the demonstration of well-regulated conduct and acceptance of group discipline over a period of several years. Candidates were required to swear oaths to accept the discipline of the group, to remain loyal to it, and to protect its secrets. Acceptance of the candidate followed a fixed, stepwise progression.

The group's *modus vivendi* was stringently regulated by ritual—ritual bathing, ritualized eating, and ritualized worship. Study of its scriptures was pursued daily, especially on the Sabbath. Many of these scriptures were idiosyncratic interpretations that served the group's own interests.

For most of its history, the sect remained exclusively male, prohibiting marriage and demanding celibacy. It renewed itself by accepting as candidates for membership the children of others. Some evidence exists that marriage was permitted at a relatively late date in the sect's history. One Qumran text graphically described the seductive women who attempted to lead righteous men astray (Broshi 1983).

A profile of the conduct and attitudes of the ideal member can be reconstructed from the scriptures. He had broken his ties with his family and replaced them with ties to the fraternity. He hated those outside his society and harbored wishes for their violent destruction. That is, his uncritical love of his new associates was purchased at the price of critical rejection of others.

He was concerned with all kinds of purity. While some of these concerns followed biblical rules, they were usually greatly elaborated. Purity of body and spirit required separation from women and lustful thoughts, ritual separation from excrement, and ritual bathing. Contempt for the impurity of others complemented the member's concern for his own purity. He conducted himself in an abstemious and self-denying manner. Subordinating himself to the discipline of the group, he had to forgo the satisfaction of personal achievement.

Reference to the problem of dealing with the mental deviant, the stupid, and the insane suggests that the sect attracted individuals who were not able to conform to demands of the outside society.

Sectarian Beliefs

Mystical and apocalyptic interests were encouraged by the promotion of certain beliefs: Special enlightenment was achieved by mystical communion with God and by pursuing the life of purity, fraternity, and abstemiousness required by the group. The communion guaranteed the authenticity of the group's beliefs as well as God's special protection. By going into the desert the group identified itself with the desert generation of Jews who had escaped from Egypt. Consequently they were destined to become the new Israel by virtue of their covenant with God. (It should be noted, however, that going into the desert was also an effective way of escaping persecution by their political enemies.) Truth could only be ascertained by reinterpreting classical scriptures in the light of the group's new insights. Sooner rather than later, the struggle between good and evil—light and darkness—would terminate with the victory of the former and the destruction of the latter. Only members of the brotherhood would survive. Though congruent with Greek and Persian antecedents, this dualistic concept was foreign to Jewish tradition and belief.

Psychodynamics

A syndrome can be reconstructed as follows: 1) There was an abdication of striving to succeed in the wider world, that is to surpass contemporaries, to win a female partner and beget children, and to acquire possessions. 2) There was a hostile rejection of the outside world and redirection of affection to other sect members. 3) There was submission to the will of God, the discipline of the sect, and to the governance of the elders and the community. 4) There was self-sacrifice and rigorous self-control: sexual desire was suppressed; physical and spiritual purity were maintained; and hard work and fulfilling a broad range of ritual obligations were demanded.

As a reward, the subject acquired the feeling of being loved and protected by the group and the leader, identified himself with the other members—feeling at one with them, acquired the sense of being loved and protected by God and having a special communion with Him, acquired the illusion that in cutting himself off from his family, sex, ambition, and personal fulfillment—in effect by destroying his real world, he would be reborn in some physical or spiritual sense. He suppressed his instinctual demands in order to comply with the demands of the superego.

In most circumstances, the performance of ritual signifies submission, and it earns a sense of gratification. Abstinence and purity secure a sense of mystical knowledge of God and intimacy with him. Thought and behavior are reconciled with conscience, so that the believer feels reconciled with parents, or at least with ultimate, transcendental parents, and enjoys the prospect that the group will defeat the establishment. Victory will be achieved vicariously through the group.

Classical apocalypse first appeared at roughly the same time as these sects. It presents a view of world history that anticipates a world destroying conflict between good and evil and the subsequent rebirth of the world. The rebirth is usually ushered in with the help of a messianic figure. The sequence of world destruction followed by rebirth is often seen at the beginning of a schizophrenic attack and with the recurrent psychotic episodes of borderline personalities. In these instances, the apocalyptic dynamic results from the effort to dissipate an impotent fury that overwhelms the patient. Presumably, public apocalypses were also intended to provide a discharge channel for an infuriated society, helpless to rid itself of the source of its pain.

The apocalyptic features in these scriptures testify that the members were united by an initial sense of impotent fury which the group helped control. Other evidence of aggressive impulses includes the hatred for the outside world, the reactive demand for love within the group, the stringency of the self-discipline, and the severity of the punishments. The rage may have arisen from individual psychopathology or in response to the actual misery of the community. Whatever the source, people were attracted to the group because it too was obsessed with rage and possessed a method for managing it.

Sects and Cults

Can we learn anything from this example of religious deviance that will aid us in understanding current cult phenomena? These groups differ from those currently active in the Western world in two important respects. They persisted for some three and a half centuries. Most of the cults with which we are concerned have been active for only a brief time—at most, decades. In addition, these ancient groups were oriented toward the beliefs and practices from which they grew. They probably absorbed some features of the religions of neighboring people. Nevertheless, they saw themselves as conservative and oriented toward the central core of Judaism in creed, ritual, and conduct. In contrast, most—though not all—current cults are outwardly oriented, incorporating religions that are alien to the local scene and to the religions in which the members were raised.

Yet on closer examination, the sects we have described above and the contemporary cults appear to have more in common. Most current religious ferment consists of alterations in the practices of religious groups that have achieved establishment status, groups that have endured for a long time and have provisions for the orderly succession of leadership. Revisions usually include changing the form of worship in the direction of greater emotional involvement with relatively less concern for philosophical issues.

Customarily there is a change in emphasis, on a renewal of older forms of worship rather than radical innovation.

Some of the groups that have been active in this way have been competing for young people who are looking for a religious structure within which they can find protection. The Lubavitch Hassidic group mentioned earlier is doing precisely that. They offer a structured organization in which acceptance is based upon compliance with traditional ritual and law, while ambition, courage, and superior achievement are considered irrelevant.

Such sects must be distinguished from cults of recent origin that possess no tested organization and have not provided for regular succession of leadership, groups that orient themselves outward toward alien creeds and standards of personal conduct. However, both types of cult are active at this time. We may speculate that the ancient Judaean sect considered here may have occupied one end of the spectrum with centrifugal groups at the other end. The fact that there are only hints of the others in ancient times may be explained by this group's greater success and endurance. A full picture of this kind of heterodox religious activity should include both centripetal and centrifugal elements.

Religion as a Solution

If that conclusion is correct, what does it tell us about the mass pursuit of religious solutions? If one looks for problems besetting the ancient world during the century and a half before and after the Christian era, any number can be found. These included economic hardships aggravated by oppressive taxation, discontent resulting from military threat or defeat, and injustice and uncertainty caused by political intrigue. Such problems abound in many places and at many times. What specifically generates a pursuit of religious solutions is probably something different.

The effective factor might be suggested by the dichotomous solutions proposed here—centripetal and centrifugal. The Hellenization that followed Alexander's conquest and the Romanization three centuries later mixed populations and created an impressive degree of cultural conflict. To quote Baron (1952):

> In that most syncretistic age of all recorded history, millions of Jews were thrown into the whorl of facile synthesis of the most disparate religious doctrines and rituals. While the corrosive forces of Hellenism had long been undermining the well-established creeds and

cultures of the Orient, growing political and economic conformity
tended to integrate the elements into a new unity.

New religious solutions were sought because the old religious
solutions had been undermined by the seductive attractions of
competing cultures.

The Maccabean War, ostensibly waged against the Seleucid
invaders, may be more correctly viewed as a civil war between
Jewish Hellenizers and Jewish religious conservatives (Bickerman
1947). About that time the Essenes and similar sects retreated to
rural and desert communities. Subsequently this conflict found less
polarized expression in the appearance of the rival Sadducee and
Pharisee parties. The Essenes represented one pole of this sectarian
conflict, while probably large numbers of other religious group-
ings, syncretistic and even more heretical, represented the other
pole. Faced with the intrusion of alien people and alien cultures,
the former group responded with religious xenophobia and the
latter with religious xenophilia.

One may guess that these groups supplied for their adherents
what each desired—a reliable, protecting, and familiar universe.
The intrusion of alien cultures changed the society's aspect by
introducing unfamiliar gods and unfamiliar expectations. Evi-
dently young people growing into adulthood in a society with such
a confusing array of models of the universe found it difficult to
commit themselves to the models that had traditionally served
their ancestors. Some were able to live with this ambiguity, finding
adequate comfort in traditional forms. Others, however, required
a more stringent, unambiguous, reliably rigid mode. Whether
young people selected the model purporting to be an authentic
representation of the origins of the tradition or the model that
offered the promise of the unfamiliar was determined by the
dynamics of the believer's relation with their parents and community.

In our current dilemma, many of our youth require the certainty of a unique protecting universe. They cannot tolerate the
ambiguity of a pluralistic community, and they are attracted by
religious groups that promise to fill their needs. Whether they
select a centripetally oriented or a centrifugally oriented group is
determined among other factors by the resolution of their childhood conflicts with parents and problems of self-esteem.

The intolerance of ambiguity and the quest for certainty
reflect the lack of confidence, the timidity, the low self-esteem, and
the polarization of attitudes and loyalties that usually accompany

various personality disorders. How disordered the personality has to be to require such a restrictive external structure depends on how far the traditional universe has disintegrated, how shaken are the supports and protection it offers, and how seriously challenged it is by alien, alternate universes. We do not know whether the incidence of personality disorders has fluctuated over time. *A priori*, there is no reason to believe the incidence fluctuates at all, though it may well be influenced by factors such as nutrition and modes of child rearing.

The Need for Certainty

In any case, there is a challenge to the youth of today that is similar to that offered to the youth of Judea two millennia ago. Aliens have been introduced into most large Western communities not by invading armies but by facile communication, rapid translation, television and movies, and easy travel. Traditional local forms vie with alternatives. Cosmopolitanism has brought with it a tolerance of dissent as well and with it a breakdown of traditional hierarchies and hierarchical values. That breakdown has facilitated both vertical and horizontal mobility, and this involves a challenge to young people to rise above the status of their parents. It is consistent with our observations that the youth who are most fearful of competition, making choices, and fulfilling responsibilities seek the security of an apparently noncompetitive fraternity that protects them from the harsh, unfriendly universe that the rest of us inhabit.

Apocalyptic elements can be found in modern cults, similar to those described in the Dead Sea sects. Jonestown, for instance, destroyed itself in an apocalyptic suicide. But even when these elements are not present, there is evidence of barely controlled fury, usually complemented by exaggerated professions of love within the group. Infuriated by their fear of making their way in a relatively unstructured society, some young people will find cults attractive, offering them a sense of rebirth into a loving fraternity— a kind of infinitely loving, understanding, embracing mother. Chasseguet-Smirgel (1985) has described the maternal quality of such groups and has seen the messianic group leader as a guide rather than a father.

We all require a sense of the predictability if not the benignity of the world that we inhabit. When inner discontent or external challenge destroys that image, most of us seek a substitute source of certainty. Involvement in cults or sects is one way of addressing this need. Those who require a literal structure promising restoration of what has been lost may find it either in a sectarian renewal of the origins of one's own tradition or in cultic involvement in form of worship that are exotic and have not yet been sources of disappointment.

References

Baron S: A Social and Religious History of the Jews. Vol II. New York, Columbia University, 1952

Betz O: Dead sea scrolls, in The Interpreters Dictionary of the Bible. Edited by Buttrick GA.Nashville, TN, Abingdon, 1962

Bickerman E: From Ezra to the Last of the Maccabees. New York, Schocken Books, 1947

Broshi M: Beware the wiles of the wanton woman. Biblical Archaeological Review IX(4):54–56, 1983

Burrows M: The Dead Sea Scrolls. New York, Viking, 1954

Chasseguet-Smirgel J: The Ego Ideal. New York, WW Norton, 1985

Farmer WR Essenes, in The Interpreters Dictionary of the Bible. Edited by Buttrick GA. Nashville, TN, Abingdon, 1962

Gaster TH (trans): The Dead Sea Scriptures. Garden City, NY, Anchor Books, 1964

Josephus: The Jewish War. Translated by Williamson GA. Harmondsworth, Middlesex, Penguin Books, 1959

Licht J: Dead Sea sect, in Encyclopedia Judaica. Edited by Roth C, Wigoder G. Jerusalem, Encyclopedia Judaica Press, 1972

Chapter 7

Suggestions for Therapists and Parents

As noted in the Preface, The Committee undertook this study because of widespread uneasiness with the increasing prevalence of new cults and fears about their influence on youth. Parents expressed anger and hurt over children who had deserted, ignored, and scorned them. They also expressed legitimate concern about their children's well-being. Because of the widely accepted notion that those who join cults are "brainwashed," the practice of kidnapping and "deprogramming" cult members has been employed, often with unhappy emotional results, certainly with questionable legal justification. Some judges have approved the seizure of these youth. Other decisions have supported the member's right to remain in his cult, and in fact, have upheld claims against parents accused of kidnapping their offspring. In any case, we need to question whether "exit counselling" that is harsh, involuntary, and possibly illegal, can be of any benefit to parent or child.

Deprogramming, or some other more benign form of involuntary treatment might be considered appropriate if the subject is clearly psychotic. In that circumstance, it is possible to obtain legal sanction through the use of guardianships or conservatorships. But we have pointed out that psychosis is not common among cult members. Psychotic individuals do not make good adherents and are usually not welcome. Similarly, cult leaders, while they may be grandiose, are rarely psychotic. If a charismatic leader were to show evidence of psychosis, or seem clearly intent on and capable of leading a cult into an orgy of self-destruction and murder, most would agree that unsolicited intervention would be justified. The

47

law has on occasion decided in favor of parents who involuntarily removed children from cults where there was legitimate question of the members' safety. On the other hand, if a guru wished to acquire a Rolls Royce for each day of the year and his well-to-do and apparently sane adherents wished to accommodate him, should the law be called in, provided no illegal acts were being committed? After all, freedom of choice is a valuable asset in our society. It should also be kept in mind that newspaper and magazine reports about cults tend to be slanted, restricted to those in which sexual orgies, cruel treatment, extortion, and other misdeeds are committed. A cult or cult leader who is helpful and caring is not newsworthy.

The Question of Brainwashing

Does the accusation of brainwashing hold up? That depends on how we define the term. Originally, the term "brainwashing" was applied to prisoners of war, detained in isolation from compatriots, treated harshly, and at the same time indoctrinated into the cause of the enemy who had total control over them. While this rarely, if ever, happens in the induction of cult members, it might be argued that forced isolation from family and friends predisposes "captive" recruits to identification with the cult's leadership and goals. When the term is used more loosely, we run into obvious problems. We might include the manipulations of public relations experts, advertising agencies, the power of well-financed political campaigns, and the work of missionaries. Eileen Barker, a sociologist and Dean of Undergraduate Studies at the London School of Economics, has written a comprehensive sociological study of the Moonies following a year's sojourn with them: *The Making of a Moonie: Choice or Brainwashing?* (Barker 1984). She maintains that brainwashing is not used to induce members to join that group. "There is no evidence that any kind of physical coercion is used by the Moonies, or that the diet or workshop activities seriously impair the biological functioning of the guests to the extent that they would be judged incapable of behaving 'normally. . . .' To her mind, personal involvement is fostered principally through the experience of a loving, caring community.

Indoctrination at an early age is no doubt the most important means of gaining adherents to any faith, established or eccentric. As we have seen, children brought up within well-structured religious communities rarely join cults. Rational judgement has little to do with any religious affiliation; indoctrination of those with a need to belong has a lot to do with it.

Reasons for Joining

Our investigations suggest that youths join cults because they sense a void in their lives. Consciously or unconsciously, they feel alienated from their parents and their society. Often they are driven by anxiety and depression, although they may be only dimly aware of it. They do not feel at home in the adult world and they fear they are incapable of carrying on independently. They seek someone, often a loving parent or big brother, who promises to take care of them, to replace what they perceive to be a stern, unloving parent, or one who has proffered no guidelines to live by. They seek a safe protecting environment among others of a similar disposition who will band together against the outside world.

Such wishes are not actually unusual among youth and do not in and of themselves indicate serious emotional problems. They are part of the developmental process—part of growing up. All of us, but especially adolescents and young adults experience some conflict between adult aspirations and regressive longings for childhood. Many believe that the process of growth requires the adolescent to exaggerate, at least temporarily, the distance between himself and his parents. This is the period when young people become most fervently involved in any number of righteous causes and develop intense idealizing attachments to friends and to adults outside of the family, such as teachers and coaches, or even more superficially to movie stars and rock musicians. Common too is the need to conform one's behavior and appearance to the arbitrary standards of the peer group. This is the period of fads in food, clothing, aesthetics, and even thought. Many developmental theorists see this behavior as a kind of experimentation, a trying on of different roles and identifications, removed from parents, but still within the protective bounds of wider society, to the end of developing a unique personal identity.

For the youth who is particularly helpless, dependent, or incompetent, these options for "normative" rebellion are unavailable. The young person who has not previously achieved a sufficiently stable sense of self-esteem or social presence will not be able to work industriously toward any goals; nor will he be able to form the attachments needed to withstand the emotional chaos that inevitably accompanies hormonal upheaval and radical social experimentation. In this case, the cult presents an attractive, if ultimately unrewarding, alternative. As we have seen, membership can provide mentors, goals, and ideals; supervisors to help contain impulses; a group with which to identify; routine to assist in achieving industry; and even a place to live; while it demands very little in return. Through joining, a "psychosocial moratorium" can be effected and in some more fortunate instances, this quiescent period can be used in the service of true developmental progress.

Unfortunately, it is more often the case that cult pressures prevent personality integration. The cult pressures encourage infantilism and discourage individuality and independence. Thus, the cults tend to aggravate rather than resolve the underlying problems that caused the youth to join, even though he or she may achieve subjective relief from loneliness and depression, and behavioral control over aggressive, addictive, or self-destructive impulses so long as he or she remains within the group.

Advice to Therapists and to Families of Cult Members

Inasmuch as the initial request for treatment will most likely come from the parents of cult members, our immediate response will be directed to their needs. It is a difficult but crucial task to slowly detoxify the situation so that distressed parents may become more objective in their appraisals and more rational in their responses. At first, patient listening may be all that can be done. Hopefully, this stage will lead to some clarification of the parents' intention in seeking treatment. It is of utmost importance that the therapist not be moved by the family's urgency to state opinions before he or she has had the chance to learn the facts, or to offer his or her services in legal disputes or involuntary treatment before it is certain that such services are warranted. In virtually all cases, it will be necessary to have some direct contact with the cult member before offering judgements as to his or her sanity, competency, or well-being. To act otherwise, based on indirect information or personal reaction would be to abuse one's claim to professional expertise.

Though it is possible to make many generalizations about the religious cults, the fact remains that for any given individual, joining is a complex process with many determinants. The clinician must evaluate many diverse variables in order to reach an understanding of a particular case. These involve not only the individual's personality and developmental processes, but also the nature of the specific cult and its dynamics. The cult member's family and even the cultural influence of his or her social milieu need to be considered.

Understanding the Cult Member

Most parents will be acutely afraid of losing all contact with their children. Therapists can direct initial efforts to this concern. They can remind parents that a high percentage of youths leave cults after fairly short periods, and they can point out that if a child knows that his or her family has acted reasonably and respectfully, neither overwhelming nor abandoning the individual, he or she will be more likely to eventually return to the family. This would be an appropriate time to obtain a detailed history; in concentrating on providing information about their child and his or her background, parents may feel that they are acting expeditiously and thus anxiety may be relieved without premature and ill-advised rescue operations. Talking about their child will also give parents a chance to become comfortable with the clinician before approaching more sensitive topics, such as their own relationship and other stresses within the family.

The parents' story will probably focus on the trials and tribulations of the adolescent period. Parents might be reassured that many adolescents display difficult behaviors and that this does not necessarily indicate emotional illness. Any events that parents judged to be particularly traumatic should be discussed, as well as any known history of sociopathy and difficulties with the law, of mental illness, including substance abuse, and any history of psychiatric treatment. Specific physical disabilities should be mentioned also.

Parents should describe any mental illness or relevant physical illness in family members. In screening for occult mental illness, parents should be asked whatever questions one might otherwise ask the patient directly. Were they aware of anxiety or depressive behavior? of rebelliousness? Did the child express much anger, and if so was this done in overt or more subtle ways? Was the child physically abusive toward family or friends? Was there a history of abuse by others? It would be useful to obtain some sense of the child's general personality style, for example, aggressive versus passive attitudes.

The child's social interactions should be described: What kind of relationship existed between parent and child? How many children are in the family and what was the identified patient's birth order? How did the child feel about his or her place in the family constellation? What were the child's relations with friends of the same and the opposite sex? Was he or she shy? What were his or her sexual attitudes? Was the child envious of others? Did he or she feel mistreated? Did the child seem "spoiled" or entitled?

A history of cognitive and intellectual achievement would include a discussion of school performance and estimates of intellectual potential (including specific intellectual deficiencies, if known), attitudes toward schoolwork, particular areas of proficiency, and evidence of independent initiative, such as hobbies or extracurricular activities. Was the child ambitious or lackadaisical, independent or conforming? An assessment of moral and ideological development might include a description of the child's religious background, and any expressed attitudes toward religion, politics, and world events.

Interviews with siblings and, if possible, with the individual himself or herself, would facilitate understanding. Comparison between the parents' description and direct clinical observation would be of particular interest.

Understanding the Cult

The cult should be studied from all available perspectives. While the real facts about the cult's beliefs and practices are obviously most important, the way the cult is viewed by parents and by the individual member may well be distorted or at least idiosyncratic. It would be important to be aware of this in planning a treatment approach. One could obtain a description of the group from the parents, from the youth and or from other members, from materials published by the cult itself or by outside investigators. An actual visit to the cult would be a valuable adjunct. The goal of this evaluation would be as full a description as possible of all aspects of cult membership, including the leader, the members, the beliefs, and the life-style.

Descriptions of recruiting and induction techniques might reveal evidence of "brainwashing" in its original sense, of seductive "love bombing," of forcible detention and physical or psychological terrorization.

Data on members might include demographic description and personals observations. Does behavior appear stereotyped? Are members manneristic or wearing a fixed smile? Are their opinions rigid and dogmatic, or is there room for intellectual flexibility and emotional depth? What is demanded of members? Are they free to leave the cult if they desire? What percentage do so, and over what time course? Does the cult demand absolute obedience? What happens to those who do not acquiesce? Are members humiliated or forced to perform shameful acts? Are they threatened? Are they physically or psychologically abused? Are they sexually abused? Are they well-fed and cared for? Are they permitted adequate sleep? Is the work schedule overly arduous? What is the quality of relationships within the cult? Are members infantilized to an extent that precludes maturation? Are sexual relations encouraged, and if so, to what extent does the cult attempt to control the choice of partners and the nature of the relationship? If children are born or brought into the cult, are the parents permitted to function as such or does the group take over? Are children beaten or otherwise abused? How are they educated?

Questions about the guru would include an assessment of his or her sanity and personal integrity. What is the leader's attitude toward money? Are members expected to raise funds for the group? Are they expected to turn over their personal assets and possessions? Has the group or the guru been sued, and if so, what was the issue and its outcome?

Understanding the Family of Origin

Finally, the parents and family need to be studied. Of course, much will have been learned about them in the course of the interviews. Now, gaps can be filled in. What is the character of each parent? Are they introspective, or do they seek explanations that are entirely external to themselves? Are they interested in understanding the situation at hand, or do they insist on an active "solution"? Is the need for action based entirely on guilt, anger over the child's difficult behavior, or a sense that they have been rejected? Are they self-critical or self-righteous? How do they understand the child's choice of the cult? What is the family's social and economic background? How is family life structured? What is expected of children and how are expectations communicated? Were parents either excessively strict or excessively indulgent? What is the moral and religious history? What religious rituals were observed, and what was the parental attitude toward them? What sort of behavioral and social values do parents hold, and how is the value system implemented? Did children appear to be in agreement with family attitudes and practices? Was dissent expressed, and if so was this tolerated or encouraged? What is the emotional state of the parents, and of any other children?

Recommendations

If evaluation of the cult indicates that it is not exploitative, and if the youth is both sane and satisfied for the moment in being part of it, there can hardly be good reason to exert extreme pressure on the youth to leave. If the cult is clearly abusive, making extortionate demands and forcing members into dangerous positions, legal action may be reasonable, especially if the child is a minor. As noted previously, the court has even upheld forcible removal of non-minors in situations where there is clear evidence of danger, but disagreements over what constitutes danger and the difficulty of proving such an allegation make the outcome of this course of action uncertain at best. At worst, kidnapping and involuntary treatment that fails will seriously compromise any trust that exists between parent and child, and will compound any acrimony. If action was undertaken without legal sanction, parents run the additional risk of legal judgements against them.

Discussions with the youth in which parents and psychotherapist convey a sympathetic attitude based on informed understanding may in some cases effect a changed view. But most members will not accede to parental requests that they leave the cult, even when the concern seems genuine and well founded. In these cases, parents can only hope that the maturational process will continue, and will eventually render the cult less necessary to the child so that he or she can see its shortcomings and leave of his or her own volition. If this does not happen, chances are that the cult is serving a necessary purpose for the child, however maladaptively, and nothing will be gained by attempting to intimidate the child into leaving.

When members do leave cults, the transition can be quite difficult, even for those judged to be emotionally healthy. They may feel socially isolated or cut adrift, anxious about resuming their place in the outside world. They may feel regressed, and they may exhibit all the symptoms that were present prior to joining the cult. Psychotherapy at this stage would be best kept supportive, encouraging a constructive adaptation to life, and leaving any deeper interpretive work until such time as the patient has re-achieved a sense of stability. Additionally, some patients may experience distress over traumatic aspects of their time within the cult. Therapy in this case, as with other posttraumatic disorders, should include the opportunity for review and re-telling, at the patient's own pace and free from value judgements or parental demands, so the patient may be able to master the experience in his or her own way.

Conclusion

In this report we have presented what we feel is an even-handed assessment of the current cult phenomenon from several vantage points. It is important to remember that most, if not all mainstream religions began life as cults.

Through our study, we have been able to arrive at several conclusions:

1. Cults run a spectrum from relatively benign organizations that are clearly tolerable within our laws, to extremely malignant enterprises that justify legal intervention to prevent people from joining them.
2. While we do not see membership in such groups as the best way for young people to negotiate the transition from childhood to independent adult life, we have found that in some cases, the cults have served this function.
3. Whatever the situation, the therapist confronted with a distressed family needs to proceed carefully, with circumspection and sensitivity until adequate evaluation can be made. Uninformed, rash intervention may do more harm than good.
4. In all cases, even the most dire, it is best for family members to maintain constructive dialogue with their children or siblings who are the cults' victims.

While we share the concern of many who are worried about the potentially destructive aspects of cults, we feel that the psychiatrist's actions must remain true to his or her charge as an expert in evaluation and a facilitator of emotional healing. The psychiatrist must avoid seduction by the more attractive, but ultimately less helpful, roles of "rescuer" or "judge."

GAP Committees and Membership

Committee on Adolescence

Warren J. Gadpaille, Denver, CO, *Chairperson*
Hector R. Bird, New York, NY
Ian A. Canino, New York, NY
Michael G. Kalogerakis, New York, NY
Paulina F. Kernberg, New York, NY
Clarice J. Kestenbaum, New York, NY
Richard C. Marohn, Chicago, IL
Silvio J. Onesti, Jr., Belmont, MA

Committee on Aging

Gene D. Cohen, Washington, DC, *Chairperson*
Karen Blank, West Hartford, CT
Eric D. Caine, Rochester, NY
Charles M. Gaitz, Houston, TX
Ira R. Katz, Philadelphia, PA
Andrew F. Leuchter, Los Angeles, CA
Gabe J. Maletta, Minneapolis, MN
Richard A. Margolin, Nashville, TN
George H. Pollock, Chicago, IL
Kenneth M. Sakauye, New Orleans, LA
Charles A. Shamoian, Larchmont, NY
F. Conyers Thompson, Jr., Atlanta, GA

Committee on Alcoholism and the Addictions

Joseph Westermeyer, Minneapolis, MN, *Chairperson*
Margaret H. Bean-Bayog, Lexington, MA

Susan J. Blumenthal, Washington, DC
Richard J. Frances, Newark, NJ
Marc Galanter, New York, NY
Edward J. Khantzian, Haverhill, MA
Earl A. Loomis, Jr., Augusta, GA
Sheldon I. Miller, Newark, NJ
Robert B. Millman, New York, NY
Steven M. Mirin, Belmont, MA
Edgar P. Nace, Dallas, TX
Norman L. Paul, Lexington, MA
Peter Steinglass, Washington, DC
John S. Tamerin, Greenwich, CT

Committee on Child Psychiatry

Peter E. Tanguay, Los Angeles, CA, *Chairperson*
James M. Bell, Canaan, NY
Harlow Donald Dunton, New York, NY
Joseph Fischhoff, Detroit, MI
Joseph M. Green, Madison, WI
John F. McDermott, Jr., Honolulu, HI
David A. Mrazek, Denver, CO
Cynthia R. Pfeffer, White Plains, NY
John Schowalter, New Haven, CT
Theodore Shapiro, New York, NY
Leonore Terr, San Francisco, CA

Committee on College Students

Earle Silber, Chevy Chase, MD, *Chairperson*
Robert L. Arnstein, Hamden, CT
Varda Backus, La Jolla, CA
Harrison P. Eddy, New York, NY
Myron B. Liptzin, Chapel Hill, NC
Malkah Tolpin Notman, Brookline, MA
Gloria C. Onque, Pittsburgh, PA
Elizabeth Aub Reid, Cambridge, MA
Lorraine D. Siggins, New Haven, CT
Tom G. Stauffer, White Plains, NY

Committee on Cultural Psychiatry

Ezra Griffith, New Haven, CT, *Chairperson*
Edward Foulks, New Orleans, LA
Pedro Ruiz, Houston, TX

Ronald Wintrob, Providence, RI
Joe Yamamoto, Los Angeles, CA

Committee on the Family

Herta A. Guttman, Montreal, PQ, *Chairperson*
W. Robert Beavers, Dallas, TX
Ellen M. Berman, Merrion, PA
Lee Combrinck-Graham, Evanston, IL
Ira D. Glick, New York, NY
Frederick Gottlieb, Los Angeles, CA
Henry U. Grunebaum, Cambridge, MA
Ann L. Price, Avon, CT
Lyman C. Wynne, Rochester, NY

Committee on Governmental Agencies

Roger Peele, Washington, DC, *Chairperson*
Mark Blotcky, Dallas, TX
James P. Cattell, San Diego, CA
Thomas L. Clannon, San Francisco, CA
Naomi Heller, Washington, DC
John P.D. Shemo, Charlottesville, VA
William W. Van Stone, Washington, DC

Committee on Handicaps

William H. Sack, Portland, OR, *Chairperson*
Norman R. Bernstein, Cambridge, MA
Meyer S. Gunther, Wilmette, IL
Robert Nesheim, Duluth, MN
Betty J. Pfefferbaum, Norman, OK
William A. Sonis, Philadelphia, PA
Margaret L. Stuber, Los Angeles, CA
George Tarjan, Los Angeles, CA
Thomas G. Webster, Washington, DC
Henry H. Work, Bethesda, MD

Committee on Human Sexuality

Bertram H. Schaffner, New York, NY, *Chairperson*
Paul L. Adams, Galveston, TX
Richard Frieman, New York, NY
Johanna A. Hoffman, Scottsdale, AZ
Joan A. Lang, Galveston, TX
Stuart E. Nichols, New York, NY

Harris B. Peck, New Rochelle, NY
John P. Spiegel, Waltham, MA
Terry S. Stein, East Lansing, MI

Committee on International Relations

Vamik D. Volkan, Charlottesville, VA, *Chairperson*
Robert M. Dorn, El Macero, CA
John S. Kafka, Washington, DC
Otto F. Kernberg, White Plains, NY
John E. Mack, Chestnut Hill, MA
Roy W. Menninger, Topeka, KS
Peter A. Olsson, Houston, TX
Rita R. Rogers, Palos Verdes Estates, CA
Stephen B. Shanfield, San Antonio, TX

Committee on Medical Education

Stephen C. Scheiber, Deerfield, IL, *Chairperson*
Charles M. Culver, Hanover, NH
Steven L. Dubovsky, Denver, CO
Saul I. Harrison, Torrance, CA
David R. Hawkins, Chicago, IL
Harold I. Lief, Philadelphia, PA
Carol Nadelson, Boston, MA
Carolyn B. Robinowitz, Washington, DC
Sidney L. Werkman, Washington, DC
Veva H. Zimmerman, New York, NY

Committee on Mental Health Services

W. Walter Menninger, Topeka, KS, *Chairperson*
Mary Jane England, Roseland, NJ
Robert O. Friedel, Richmond, VA
John M. Hamilton, Columbia, MD
Jose Maria Santiago, Tucson, AZ
Steven S. Sharfstein, Baltimore, MD
Herzl R. Spiro, Milwaukee, WI
William L. Webb, Jr., Hartford, CT
George F. Wilson, Somerville, NJ
Jack A. Wolford, Pittsburgh, PA

Committee on Planning and Marketing

Robert W. Gibson, Towson, MD, *Chairperson*
Allan Beigel, Tucson, AZ

Doyle I. Carson, Dallas, TX
Paul J. Fink, Philadelphia, PA
Robert S. Garber, Longboat Key, FL
Richard K. Goodstein, Belle Mead, NJ
Harvey L. Ruben, New Haven, CT
Melvin Sabshin, Washington, DC
Michael R. Zales, Quechee, VT

Committee on Preventive Psychiatry

Naomi Rae-Grant, London, Ont., *Chairperson*
Viola W. Bernard, New York, NY
Stephen Fleck, New Haven, CT
Brian J. McConville, Cincinnati, OH
David R. Offord, Hamilton, Ont.
Morton M. Silverman, Chicago, IL
Warren T. Vaughan, Jr., Portola Valley, CA
Ann Marie Wolf-Schatz, Conshohocken, PA

Committee on Psychiatry and the Community

Kenneth Minkoff, Woburn, MA, *Chairperson*
C. Knight Aldrich, Charlottesville, VA
David G. Greenfield, Guilford, CT
H. Richard Lamb, Los Angeles, CA
John C. Nemiah, Hanover, NH
Rebecca L. Potter, Tucson, AZ
John J. Schwab, Louisville, KY
John A. Talbott, Baltimore, MD
Allan Tasman, Louisville, KY
Charles B. Wilkinson, Kansas City, MO

Committee on Psychiatry and the Law

Joseph Satten, San Francisco, CA, *Chairperson*
Renee L. Binder, San Francisco, CA
J. Richard Ciccone, Rochester, NY
Carl P. Malmquist, Minneapolis, MN
Herbert C. Modlin, Topeka, KS
Jonas R. Rappeport, Baltimore, MD
Phillip J. Resnick, Cleveland, OH
William D. Weitzel, Lexington, KY

Committee on Psychiatry and Religion

Richard C. Lewis, New Haven, CT, *Chairperson*

Naleen N. Andrade, Honolulu, HI
Keith G. Meador, Nashville, TN
Abigail R. Ostow, Belmont, MA
Sally K. Severino, White Plains, NY
Clyde R. Snyder, Fayetteville, NC
Edwin R. Wallace, IV, Augusta, GA

Committee on Psychiatry in Industry

Barrie S. Greiff, Newton, MA, *Chairperson*
Peter L. Brill, Radnor, PA
Duane Q. Hagen, St. Louis, MO
R. Edward Huffman, Asheville, NC
Robert Larsen, San Francisco, CA
David E. Morrison, Palatine, IL
David B. Robbins, Chappaqua, NY
Jay B. Rohrlich, New York, NY
Clarence J. Rowe, St. Paul, MN
Jeffrey L. Speller, Cambridge, MA

Committee on Psychopathology

David A. Adler, Boston, MA, *Chairperson*
Jeffrey Berlant, Summit, NJ
John P. Docherty, Nashua, NH
Robert A. Dorwart, Cambridge, MA
Robert E. Drake, Hanover, NH
James M. Ellison, Watertown, MA
Howard H. Goldman, Potomac, MD
Anthony F. Lehman, Baltimore, MD
Kathleen A. Pajer, Pittsburgh, PA
Samuel G. Siris, Glen Oaks, NY

Committee on Public Education

Steven E. Katz, New York, NY, *Chairperson*
Jack W. Bonner, III, Asheville, NC
John Donnelly, Hartford, CT
Jeffrey L. Geller, Worcester, MA
Keith H. Johansen, Dallas, TX
Elise K. Richman, Scarsdale, NY
Boris G. Rifkin, Branford, CT
Andrew E. Slaby, Summit, NJ
Robert A. Solow, Los Angeles, CA
Calvin R. Sumner, Buckhannon, WV

Committee on Research

Robert Cancro, New York, NY, *Chairperson*
Jack A. Grebb, New York, NY
John H. Greist, Madison, WI
Jerry M. Lewis, Dallas, TX
John G. Looney, Durham, NC
Sidney Malitz, New York, NY
Zebulon Taintor, New York, NY

Committee on Social Issues

Ian E. Alger, New York, NY, *Chairperson*
William R. Beardslee, Waban, MA
Judith H. Gold, Halifax, N.S.
Roderic Gorney, Los Angeles, CA
Martha J. Kirkpatrick, Los Angeles, CA
Perry Ottenberg, Philadelphia, PA
Kendon W. Smith, Pearl River, NY

Committee on Therapeutic Care

Donald W. Hammersley, Washington, DC, *Chairperson*
Bernard Bandler, Cambridge, MA
Thomas E. Curtis, Chapel Hill, NC
Donald C. Fidler, Morgantown, WV
William B. Hunter, III, Albuquerque, NM
Roberto L. Jimenez, San Antonio, TX
Milton Kramer, Cincinnati, OH
Theodore Nadelson, Jamaica Plain, MA
William W. Richards, Anchorage, AK

Committee on Therapy

Allen D. Rosenblatt, La Jolla, CA, *Chairperson*
Gerald Adler, Boston, MA
Jules R. Bemporad, Boston, MA
Eugene B. Feigelson, Brooklyn, NY
Robert Michels, New York, NY
Andrew P. Morrison, Cambridge, MA
William C. Offenkrantz, Carefree, AZ

Contributing Members

Gene Abroms, Ardmore, PA
Carlos C. Alden, Jr., Buffalo, NY
Kenneth Z. Altshuler, Dallas, TX

Francis F. Barnes, Washington, DC
Spencer Bayles, Houston, TX
C. Christian Beels, New York, NY
Elissa P. Benedek, Ann Arbor, MI
Sidney Berman, Washington, DC
H. Keith H. Brodie, Durham, NC
Charles M. Bryant, San Francisco, CA
Ewald W. Busse, Durham, NC
Robert N. Butler, New York, NY
Eugene M. Caffey, Jr., Bowie, MD
Robert J. Campbell, New York, NY
Ian L.W. Clancey, Maitland, Ont.
Sanford I. Cohen, Coral Gables, FL
James S. Eaton, Jr., Washington, DC
Lloyd C. Elam, Nashville, TN
Joseph T. English, New York, NY
Louis C. English, Pomona, NY
Sherman C. Feinstein, Highland Park, IL
Archie R. Foley, New York, NY
Sidney Furst, Bronx, NY
Henry J. Gault, Highland Park, IL
Alexander Gralnick, Port Chester, NY
Milton Greenblatt, Sylmar, CA
Lawrence F. Greenleigh, Los Angeles, CA
Stanley I. Greenspan, Bethesda, MD
Jon E. Gudeman, Milwaukee, WI
Stanley Hammons, Lexington, KY
William Hetznecker, Merion Station, PA
J. Cotter Hirschberg, Topeka, KS
Johanna Hoffman, Scottsdale, AZ
Jay Katz, New Haven, CT
James A. Knight, New Orleans, LA
Othilda M. Krug, Cincinnati, OH
Judith Landau-Stanton, Rochester, NY
Alan I. Levenson, Tucson, AZ
Ruth W. Lidz, Woodbridge, CT
Orlando B. Lightfoot, Boston, MA
Norman L. Loux, Sellersville, PA
Albert J. Lubin, Woodside, CA
John A. MacLeod, Cincinnati, OH
Charles A. Malone, Barrington, RI
Peter A. Martin, Lake Orion, MI
Ake Mattsson, Charlottesville, VA

Alan A. McLean, Gig Harbor, WA
David Mendell, Houston, TX
Mary E. Mercer, Nyack, NY
Derek Miller, Chicago, IL
Richard D. Morrill, Boston, MA
Robert J. Nathan, Philadelphia, PA
Joseph D. Noshpitz, Washington, DC
Mortimer Ostow, Bronx, NY
Bernard L. Pacella, New York, NY
Herbert Pardes, New York, NY
Marvin E. Perkins, Salem, VA
David N. Ratnavale, Bethesda, MD
Richard E. Renneker, Pacific Palisades, CA
W. Donald Ross, Cincinnati, OH
Loren Roth, Pittsburgh, PA
Donald J. Scherl, Brooklyn, NY
Charles Shagass, Philadelphia, PA
Miles F. Shore, Boston, MA
Albert J. Silverman, Ann Arbor, MI
Benson R. Snyder, Cambridge, MA
David A. Soskis, Bala Cynwyd, PA
Jeanne Spurlock, Washington, DC
Brandt F. Steele, Denver, CO
Alan A. Stone, Cambridge, MA
Perry C. Talkington, Dallas, TX
Bryce Templeton, Philadelphia, PA
Prescott W. Thompson, Portland, OR
John A. Turner, San Francisco, CA
Gene L. Usdin, New Orleans, LA
Kenneth N. Vogtsberger, San Antonio, TX
Andrew S. Watson, Ann Arbor, MI
Joseph B. Wheelwright, Kentfield, CA
Robert L. Williams, Houston, TX
Paul Tyler Wilson, Bethesda, MD
Sherwyn M. Woods, Los Angeles, CA
Kent A. Zimmerman, Menlo Park, CA
Howard Zonana, New Haven, CT

Life Members

C. Knight Aldrich, Charlottesville, VA
Robert L. Arnstein, Hamden, CT
Bernard Bandler, Cambridge, MA

Walter E. Barton, Hartland, VT
Viola W. Bernard, New York, NY
Henry W. Brosin, Tucson, AZ
John Donnelly, Hartford, CT
Merrill T. Eaton, Omaha, NE
O. Spurgeon English, Narberth, PA
Stephen Fleck, New Haven, CT
Jerome Frank, Baltimore, MD
Robert S. Garber, Longboat Key, FL
Robert I. Gibson, Towson, MD
Margaret M. Lawrence, Pomona, NY
Jerry M. Lewis, Dallas, TX
Harold I. Lief, Philadelphia, PA
Judd Marmor, Los Angeles, CA
Herbert C. Modlin, Topeka, KS
John C. Nemiah, Hanover, NH
William Offenkrantz, Carefree, NM
Mabel Ross, Sun City, AZ
Julius Schreiber, Washington, DC
Robert E. Switzer, Dunn Loring, VA
George Tarjan, Los Angeles, CA
Jack A. Wolford, Pittsburgh, PA
Henry H. Work, Bethesda, MD

Board of Directors

Officers

President
Allan Beigel
P.O. Box 43460
Tucson, AZ 85733

President-Elect
Charles Wilkinson,
600 E. 22nd Street
Kansas City, MO 64108

Secretary
Doyle I. Carson
Timberlawn Psychiatric Hospital
P.O. Box 151489
Dallas, TX 75315-1489

Treasurer
Jack W. Bonner, III
Highland Hospital
P.O. Box 1101
Asheville, NC 28802

Board Members
Judith Gold
Harvey L. Ruben
Pedro Ruiz
John Schowalter

Past Presidents
*William C. Menninger 1946-51
Jack R. Ewalt 1951-53
Walter E. Barton 1953-55
*Sol W. Ginsburg 1955-57
*Dana L. Farnsworth 1957-59
*Marion E. Kenworthy 1959-61
Henry W. Brosin 1961-63
*Leo H. Bartemeier 1963-65
Robert S. Garber 1965-67
Herbert C. Modlin 1967-69
John Donnelly 1969-71
George Tarjan 1971-73
Judd Marmor 1973-75
John C. Nemiah 1975-77
Jack A. Wolford 1977-79
Robert W. Gibson 1979-81
*Jack Weinberg 1981-82
Henry H. Work 1982-85
Michael R. Zales 1985-87
Jerry M. Lewis 1987-89
Carolyn B. Robinowitz 1989-91

*deceased

PUBLICATIONS BOARD

Chairman
C. Knight Aldrich
Health Sciences Center
Box 414
Charlottesville, VA 22908

Middlesex County College

3 9320 00089365 8

Leaders and Followers

JAN 2002

Robert L. Arnstein
Judith H. Gold
Milton Kramer
W. Walter Menninger
Robert A. Solow

Consultant
John C. Nemiah

Ex-Officio
Allan Beigel
Carolyn B. Robinowitz

CONTRIBUTORS

Abbott Laboratories
American Charitable Fund
Dr. and Mrs. Richard Aron
Mr. Robert C. Baker
Maurice Falk Medical Fund
Mrs. Carol Gold
Grove Foundation, Inc.
Miss Gayle Groves
Ittleson Foundation, Inc
Mr. Barry Jacobson
Mrs. Allan H. Kalmus
Marion E. Kenworthy—Sara
Mr. Larry Korman
McNeil Pharmaceutical
Phillips Foundation
Sandoz, Inc.
Smith Kline Beckman Corpc
Tappanz Foundation, Inc.
The Upjohn Company
van American Foundation, I
Wyeth Laboratories
Mr. and Mrs. William A. Zal

RC 321 .G7 no. 132

Leaders and followers : a
psychiatri

DATE DUE

DEC 1 8 2002

WITHDRAWN

Middlesex County College
Library. Edison, NJ 08818

Demco, Inc. 38-293